Animal Lives

Having Young

Kimberley Jane Pryor

A+

Smart Apple Media
P.O. Box 3263
Mankato, MN, 56002

First published in 2010 by
MACMILLAN EDUCATION AUSTRALIA PTY LTD
15–19 Claremont St, South Yarra, Australia 3141

Visit our web site at www.macmillan.com.au or go directly to www.macmillanlibrary.com.au

Associated companies and representatives throughout the world.

Library of Congress Cataloging-in-Publication Data

Pryor, Kimberley Jane.
Having young / by Kimberley Jane Pryor.
p. cm. — (Animal lives)
Includes index.
Summary: "Gives information on ways animals reproduce and highlights different animals, both large and small from land to sea"—Provided by publisher.
ISBN 978-1-59920-403-1 (library binding)
1. Reproduction—Juvenile literature. 2. Sexual behavior in animals—Juvenile literature.
3. Animals—Juvenile literature. I. Title.
QP251.5.P79 2012
612.6—dc22
2010046005

Publisher: Carmel Heron
Managing Editor: Vanessa Lanaway
Editor: Paige Amor and Georgina Garner
Proofreader: Tim Clarke
Designer: Ben Galpin
Page layout: Ben Galpin
Photo researcher: Lesya Bryndzia (management: Debbie Gallagher)
Illustrator: Ben Spiby
Production Controller: Vanessa Johnson

Manufactured in the United States of America by Corporate Graphics
North Mankato, Minnesota
April 2011

Acknowledgements
The author and the publisher are grateful to the following for permission to reproduce copyright material:

Front cover photograph of female orang-outang and baby, courtesy of iStockphoto.com/Jason Krzyzanowski.

Nigel Dennis/ANTPhoto, **16**; Rudie Kuiter/ANTPhoto, **22**; Fredy Mercay/ANTPhoto, **4**; Murray Price/ANTPhoto, **23**; Cyril Webster/ANTPhoto, **15**; John Lewis/Auscape, **5**; Michael & Patricia Fogden/Corbis, **21**; Eric and David Hosking/Corbis, **30**; Norbert Wu/Science Faction/Corbis, **12**; iStockphoto.com/John Frink, **18**; iStockphoto.com/Jason Krzyzanowski, **24**; iStockphoto.com/Martin Ramsay, **28**; iStockphoto.com/stevenleejohnson, **14**; iStockphoto.com/Boris Tarasov, **9**; iStockphoto.com/Roger Whiteway, **26**; JupiterImages Unlimited/Photos.com, **25**; Photolibrary/Age Fotostock/Morales Morales, **10**; Photolibrary/Kevin Aitken, **8**; Photolibrary/Animals Animals/Zigmund Leszczynski, **11**; Photolibrary/Photo Researchers/Edward Kinsman, **13**; Photolibrary/Photo Researchers/Karl H Switak, **19**; Shutterstock/EcoPrint, **29**; Shutterstock/John Marquess, **20**; Shutterstock/David Nagy, **27**; Shutterstock/Steffen Foerster Photography, **17**.

The author would also like to acknowledge the following sources for information used in this book:
Coral and surgeonfish: Sigmun Lloyd, Great Barrier Reef Marine Park Authority, Pierre Gilles, Musée Océanographique de Monaco and Richard L. Klobuchar, Jr., University of Hawaii, Waikiki Aquarium.

While every care has been taken to trace and acknowledge copyright, the publisher tenders their apologies for any accidental infringement where copyright has proved untraceable. Where the attempt has been unsuccessful, the publisher welcomes information that would redress the situation.

For Nick, Thomas and Ashley

Contents

Glossary Words

When a word is printed in **bold**, you can look up its meaning in the glossary on page 31.

Animal Lives

Animals face many challenges in their lives. From the moment they are old enough to look after themselves, they have to work hard to survive. They must search for food. They need to escape from hungry **predators**. They have to find or make safe homes so they can shelter from the weather and hide from danger.

When they become adults, animals must attract mates so they can have young. Some animals travel to faraway **breeding** grounds to have their young. After they hatch or are born, many young need to be protected and cared for until they, too, are old enough to survive on their own.

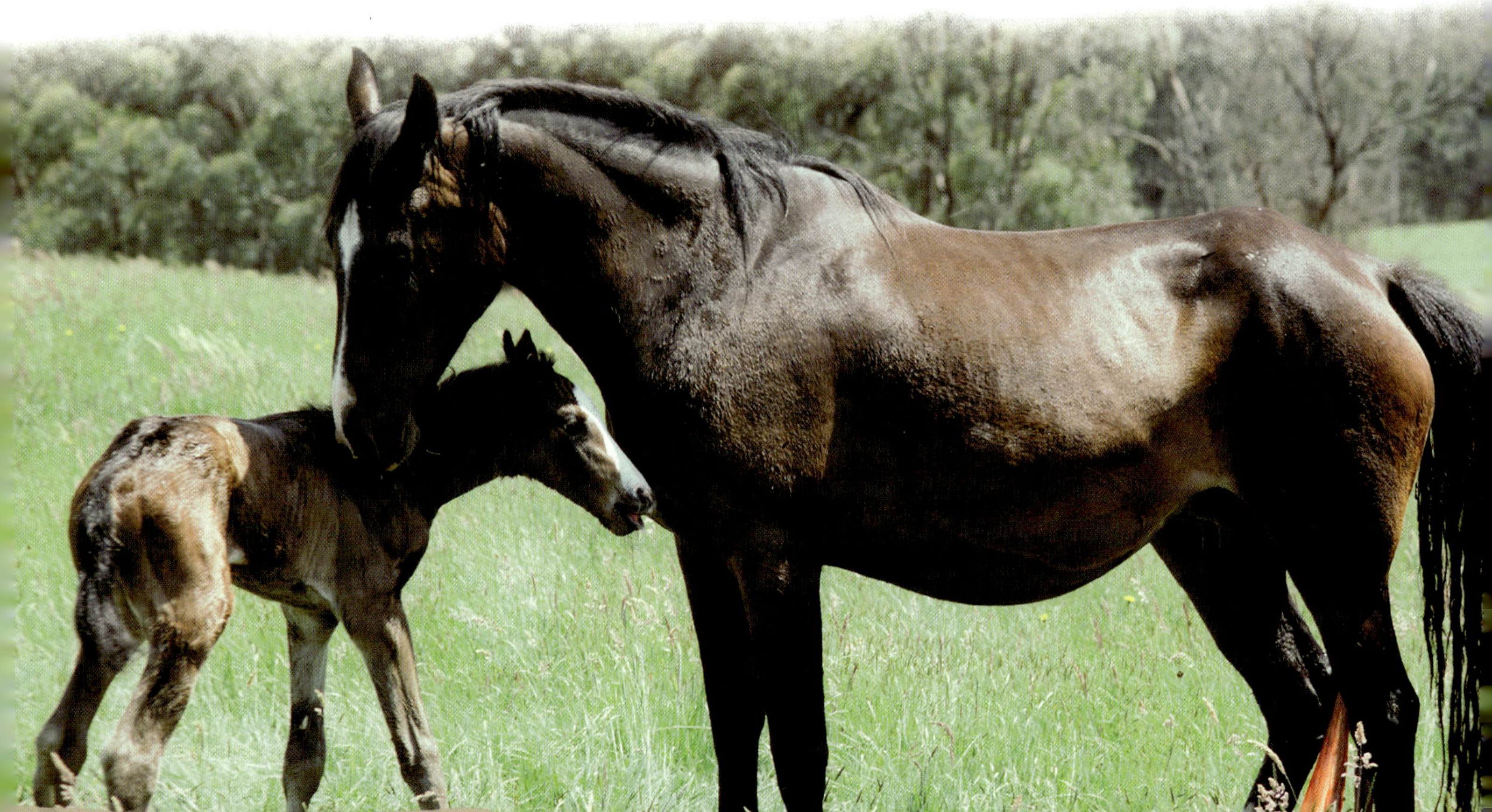

One challenge that horses face is that young horses, called foals, need to be cared for until they are old enough to care for themselves.

Having Young

Most animals grow into adults and have young. Some animals lay eggs. The eggs provide protection and food for the growing young inside them. Other animals give birth to live young. Some young can care for themselves right after hatching or being born. Other young need to be fed and protected for a period of time.

Different Ways to Have Young

Animals have young in one of two main ways. Some animals produce large numbers of eggs or young. They leave the eggs or young and go on with their own lives. Other animals produce only a few eggs or young, and they take care of them.

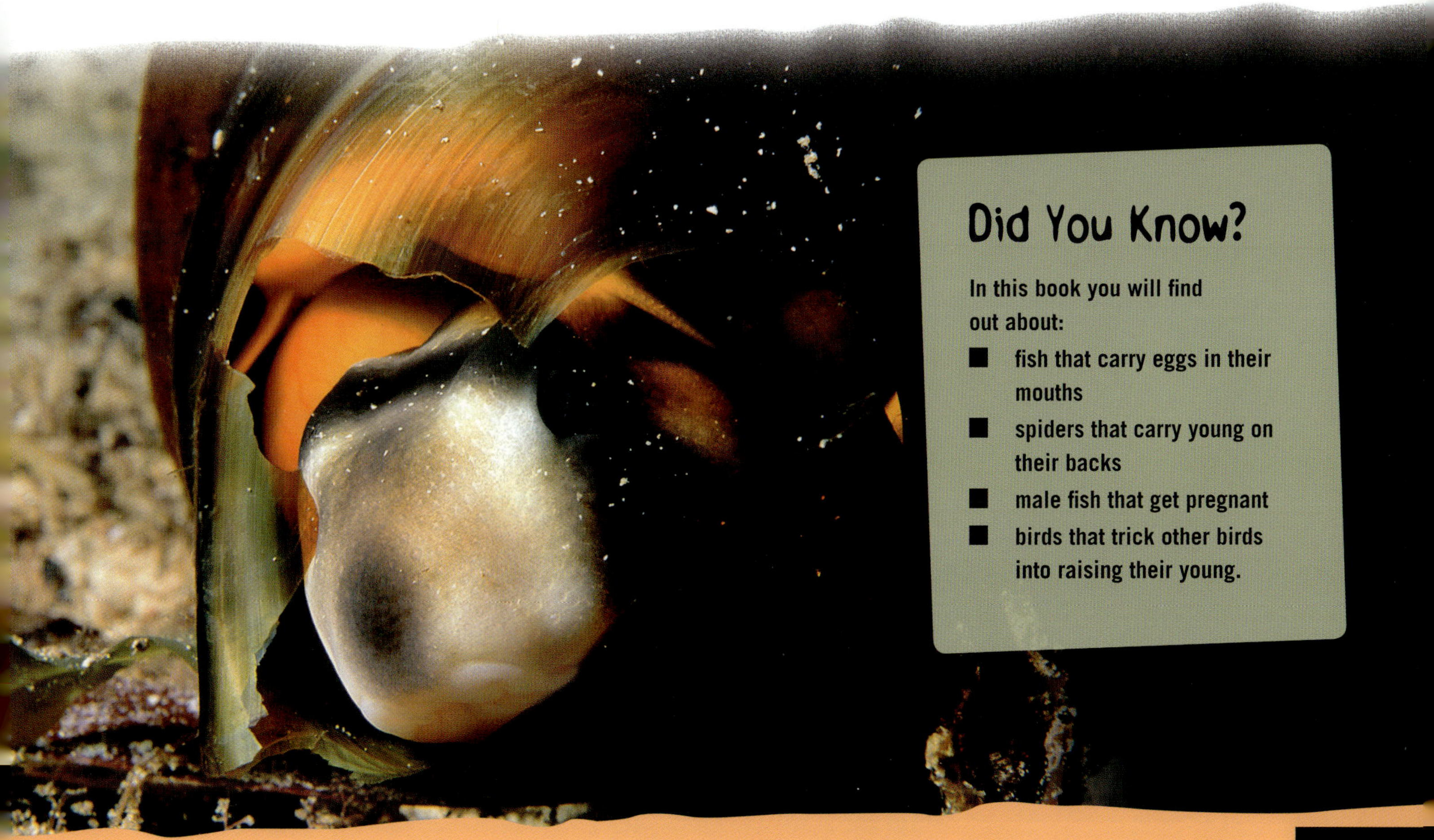

Did You Know?

In this book you will find out about:

- fish that carry eggs in their mouths
- spiders that carry young on their backs
- male fish that get pregnant
- birds that trick other birds into raising their young.

A young Port Jackson shark cares for itself right after hatching.

Virginia Opossum

A Virginia opossum is a **marsupial**. It lives for about 18 months to three years. Its young are born at a very early stage of development.

The adults breed from summer to winter. The male and female mate, and the female becomes pregnant. She has between one and three **litters** each year.

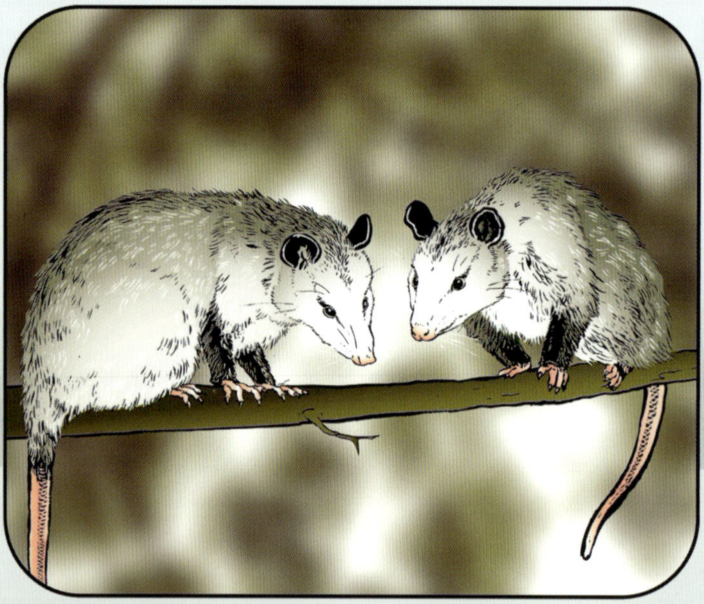

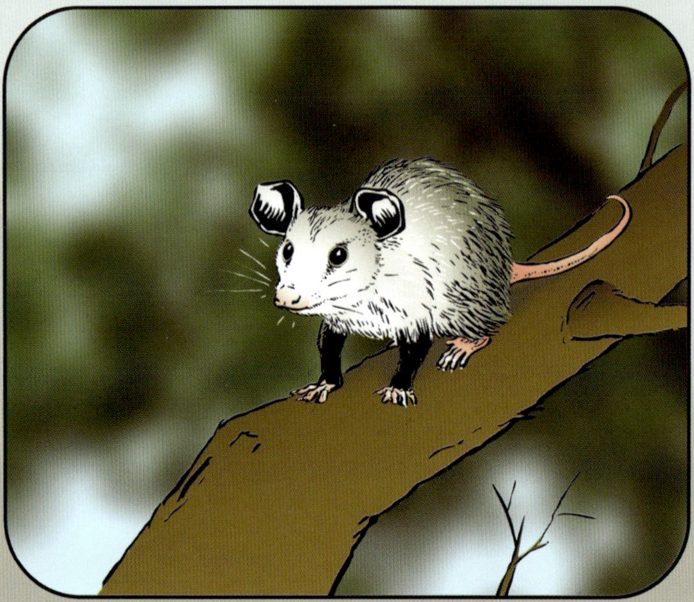

The young stop drinking milk after about three months, and they leave their mother after about five months. They are ready to breed when they are between six months and one-year old.

A life cycle is the changes an animal goes through as it grows into an adult.

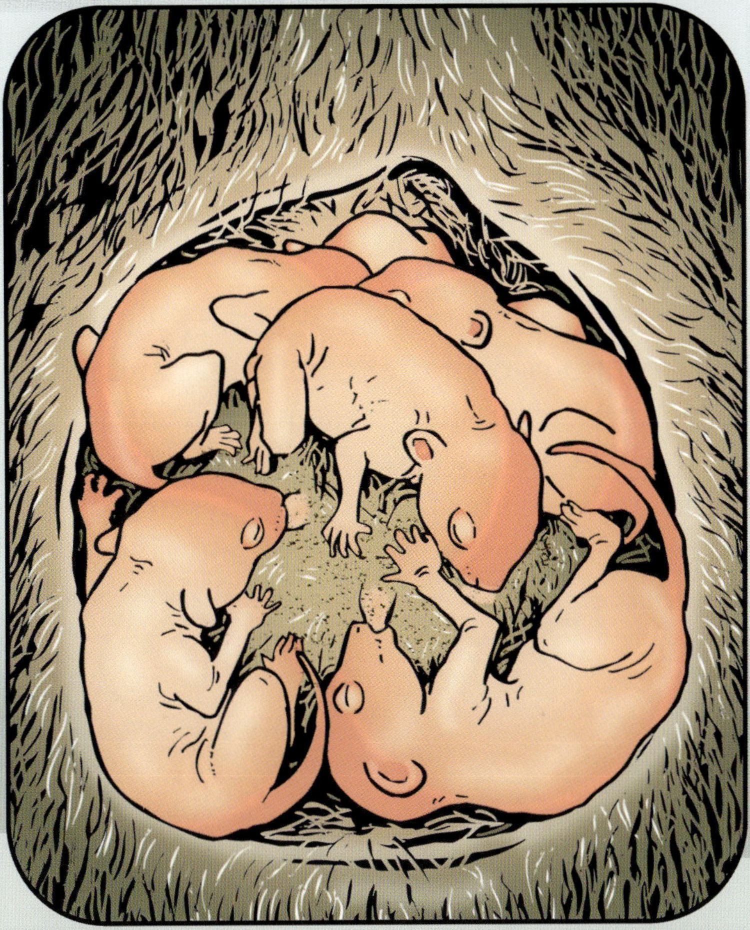

After 11 to 13 days of pregnancy, the female gives birth to about 8 young. The young crawl into their mother's pouch. Each attaches itself to a nipple and drinks its mother's milk.

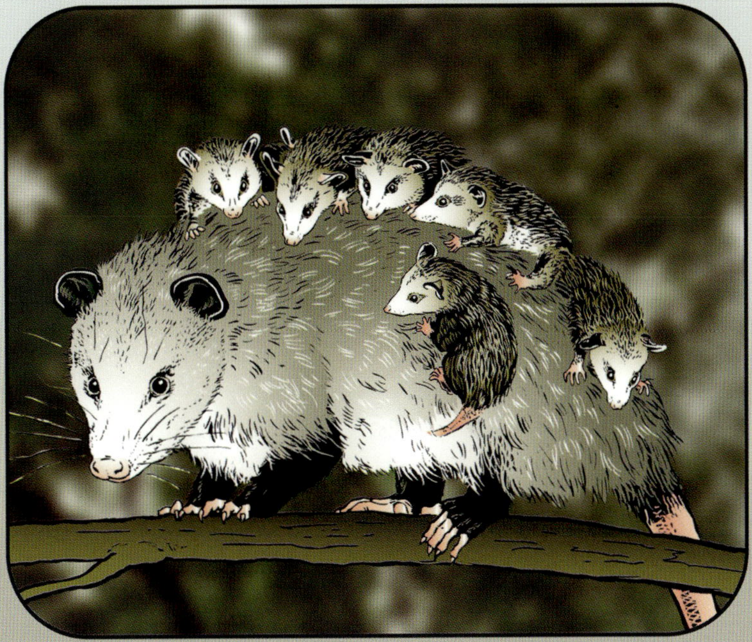

The young stay attached to the nipples for about two months. When they grow too big to fit inside the pouch, they ride on their mother's back.

Releasing Eggs and Sperm

FACT FILE

Type of Animal: invertebrate

Width: 0.04 to 9.8 inches (1–25 cm)

Habitat: hard surfaces on the ocean floor

Distribution: worldwide in seas and oceans

Number of Eggs: about 5 to 50 per coral polyp

Coral

Coral animals are called coral polyps. They release eggs and sperm into water on a warm, still night a few nights after a full moon.

Coral polyps release bundles of eggs, bundles of sperm, or bundles containing both eggs and sperm. The eggs and sperm float to the water's surface. The sperm **fertilize** the eggs. Young hatch from the eggs and swim in the water for several days or weeks. They then settle on the ocean floor and develop into coral polyps.

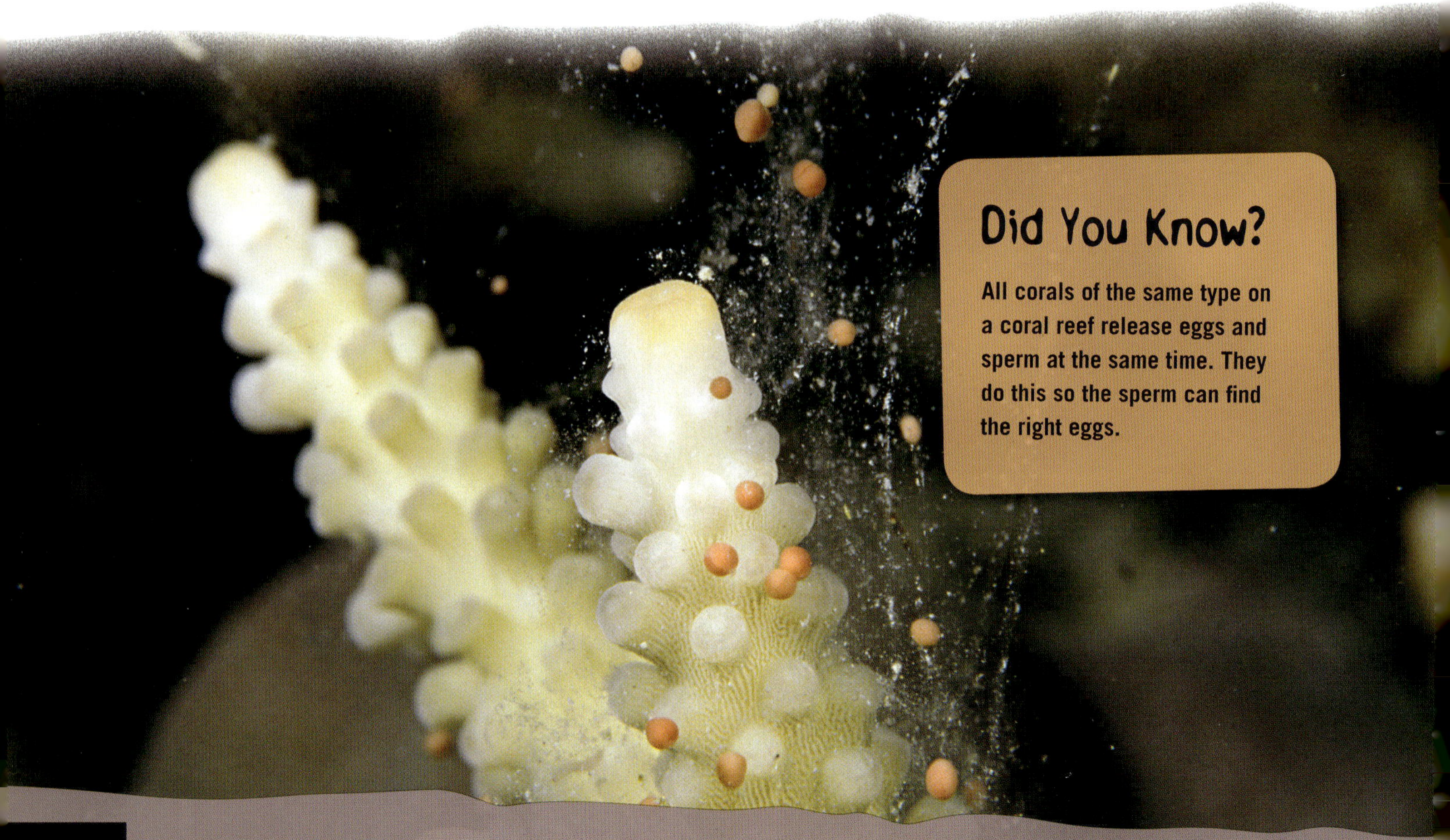

Did You Know?

All corals of the same type on a coral reef release eggs and sperm at the same time. They do this so the sperm can find the right eggs.

Some corals release orange eggs into the water.

Some animals release huge numbers of eggs and **sperm** into open water.

Surgeonfish release large numbers of eggs, because many will remain **unfertilized** or get eaten by predators.

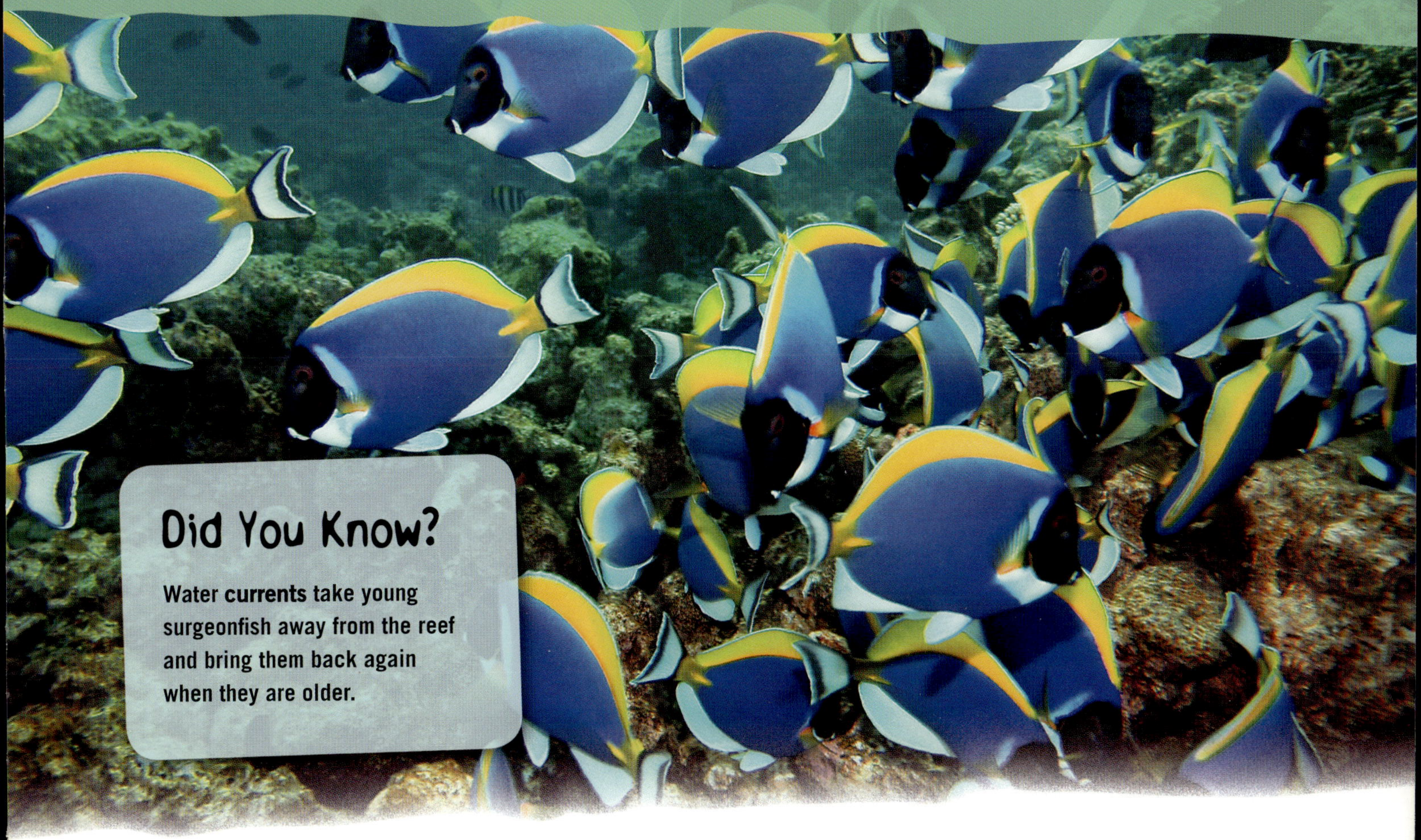

Did You Know?

Water **currents** take young surgeonfish away from the reef and bring them back again when they are older.

Surgeonfish

Surgeonfish swim to a special place on a reef edge to release eggs and sperm.

In some types of surgeonfish, a male and female rise upward and release eggs and sperm into the water. In other types, the males and females form a group, and every so often a female and several males rise above the group and release eggs and sperm into the water. The sperm fertilize the eggs. Young hatch from the eggs after about one day.

FACT FILE

Type of Animal: fish

Length: 5.9 inches to 2.5 feet (15–75 cm)

Habitat: coral and rocky reefs

Distribution: worldwide in warm seas and oceans

Number of Eggs: 50 to many hundreds per surgeonfish

Burying and Leaving Eggs

A female green turtle spends approximately three hours digging a nest and laying eggs.

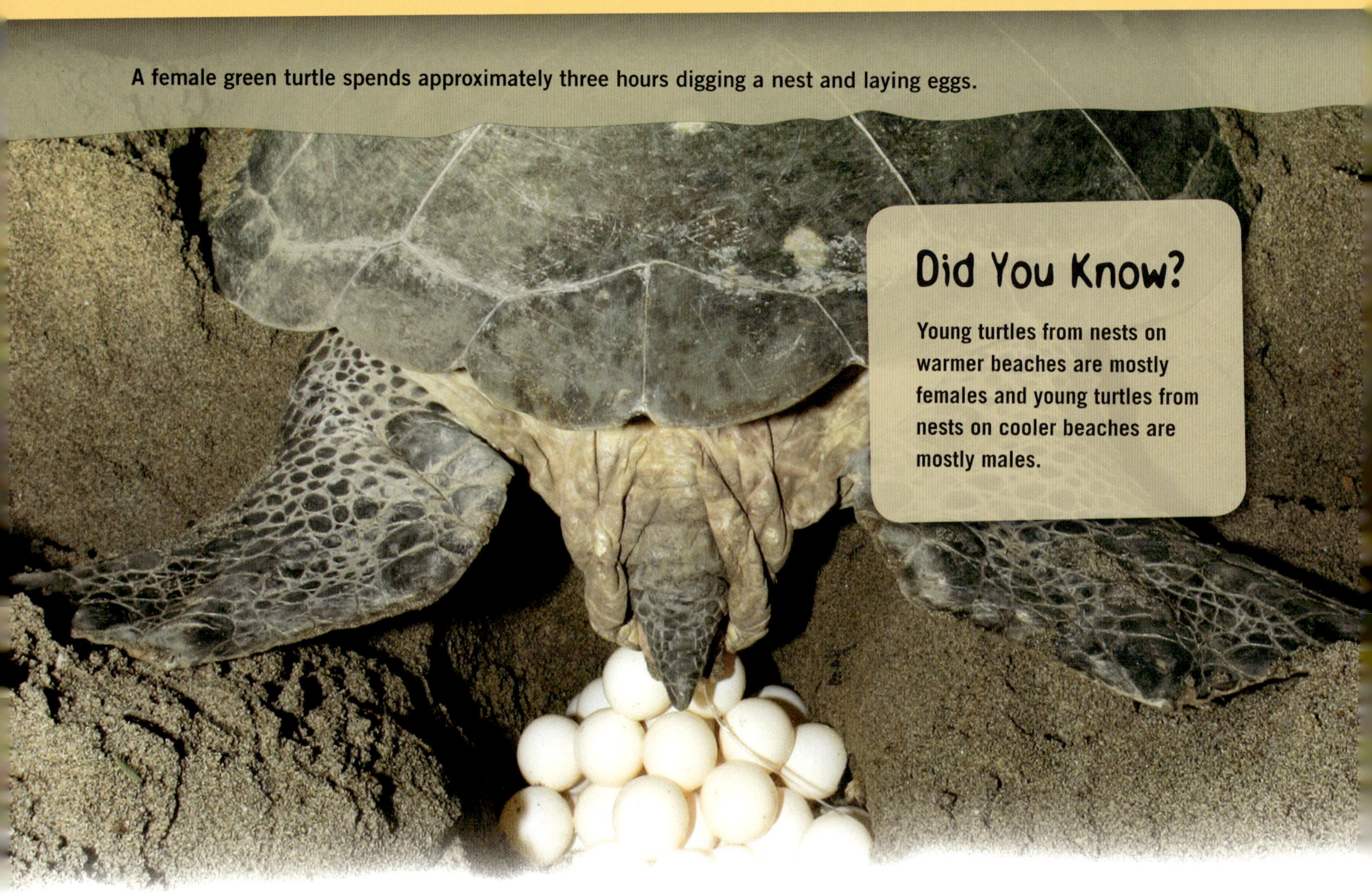

Did You Know?

Young turtles from nests on warmer beaches are mostly females and young turtles from nests on cooler beaches are mostly males.

FACT FILE

Type of Animal: reptile

Length: 3.3 feet (1 m)

Habitat: coral reefs and sea-grass beds

Distribution: Indian, Pacific, and Atlantic Oceans

Number of Eggs: approximately 120 per nest

Green Turtle

A female green turtle buries her eggs in sand. The parents do not see or care for their young.

A male and a female green turtle mate in the water. The female then drags herself onto a beach and digs a nest with her flippers. She lays her eggs in the nest and covers them with sand, before dragging herself back into the water. When the young hatch, they dig themselves out of the nest and head toward the water.

Some animals leave their eggs—but they bury them in a safe place first!

Collared Lizard

A female collared lizard buries her soft-shelled eggs in loose, sandy soil or in a burrow. The parents do not see or care for their young.

A male and a female collared lizard mate on the ground. When she is ready to lay eggs, the female digs a hole under a rock. She lays the eggs, covers them with soil, and goes away. When the young hatch, they dig themselves out of the nest and look after themselves.

FACT FILE

Type of Animal: reptile

Length: 7.8–16.5 inches (20–42 cm)

Habitat: rocky areas with few plants

Distribution: North America

Number of Eggs: 4 to 6

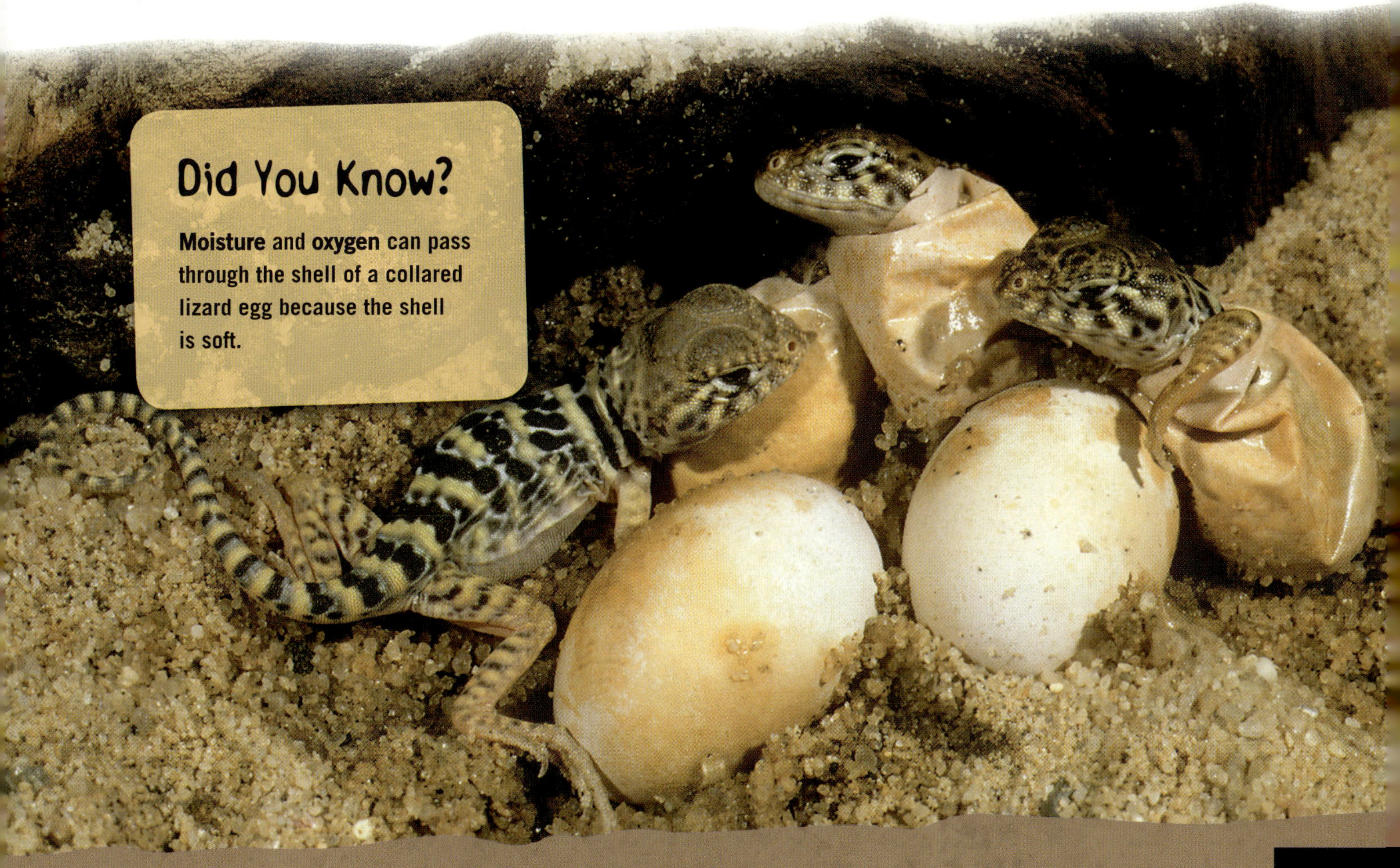

Did You Know?

Moisture and **oxygen** can pass through the shell of a collared lizard egg because the shell is soft.

Young collared lizards are on their own from the moment they hatch from their egg.

FACT FILE

Type of Animal: fish

Length: 3.9 inches to 3.7 feet (10–114 cm)

Habitat: coral reefs

Distribution: Indian, Pacific, and Atlantic Oceans

Number of Eggs: 300 to 500

Jawfish

A female jawfish lays hundreds of eggs. The male carries the eggs in his huge mouth until the young hatch.

The female jawfish follows the male jawfish into his burrow at breeding time. She lays eggs and the male fertilizes them. The male carries the fertilized eggs in his mouth for about one week. He often spits the eggs out and sucks them back in. The young hatch in his mouth and swim out into the water.

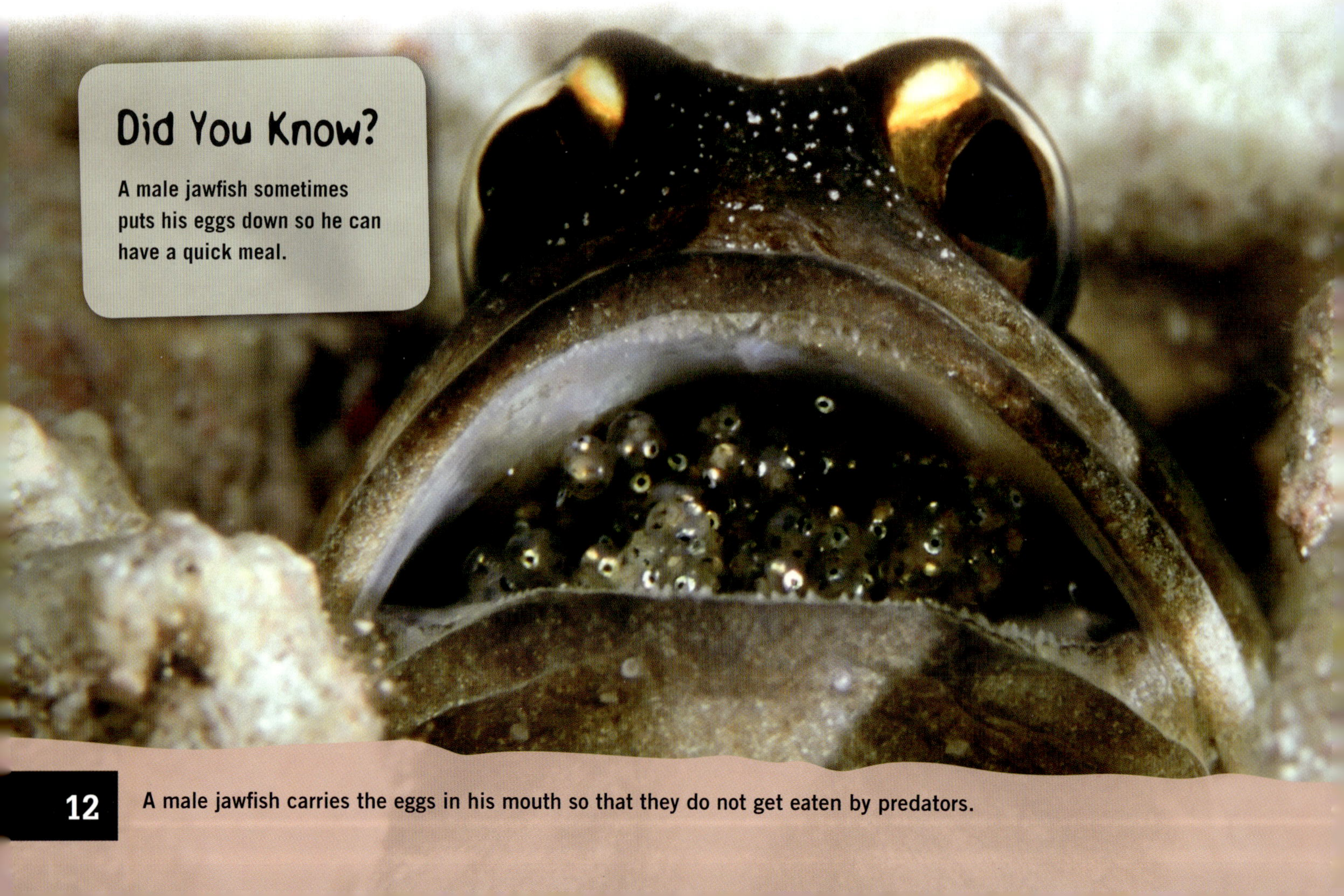

Did You Know?

A male jawfish sometimes puts his eggs down so he can have a quick meal.

A male jawfish carries the eggs in his mouth so that they do not get eaten by predators.

Animals that carry their precious eggs can protect the eggs from danger.

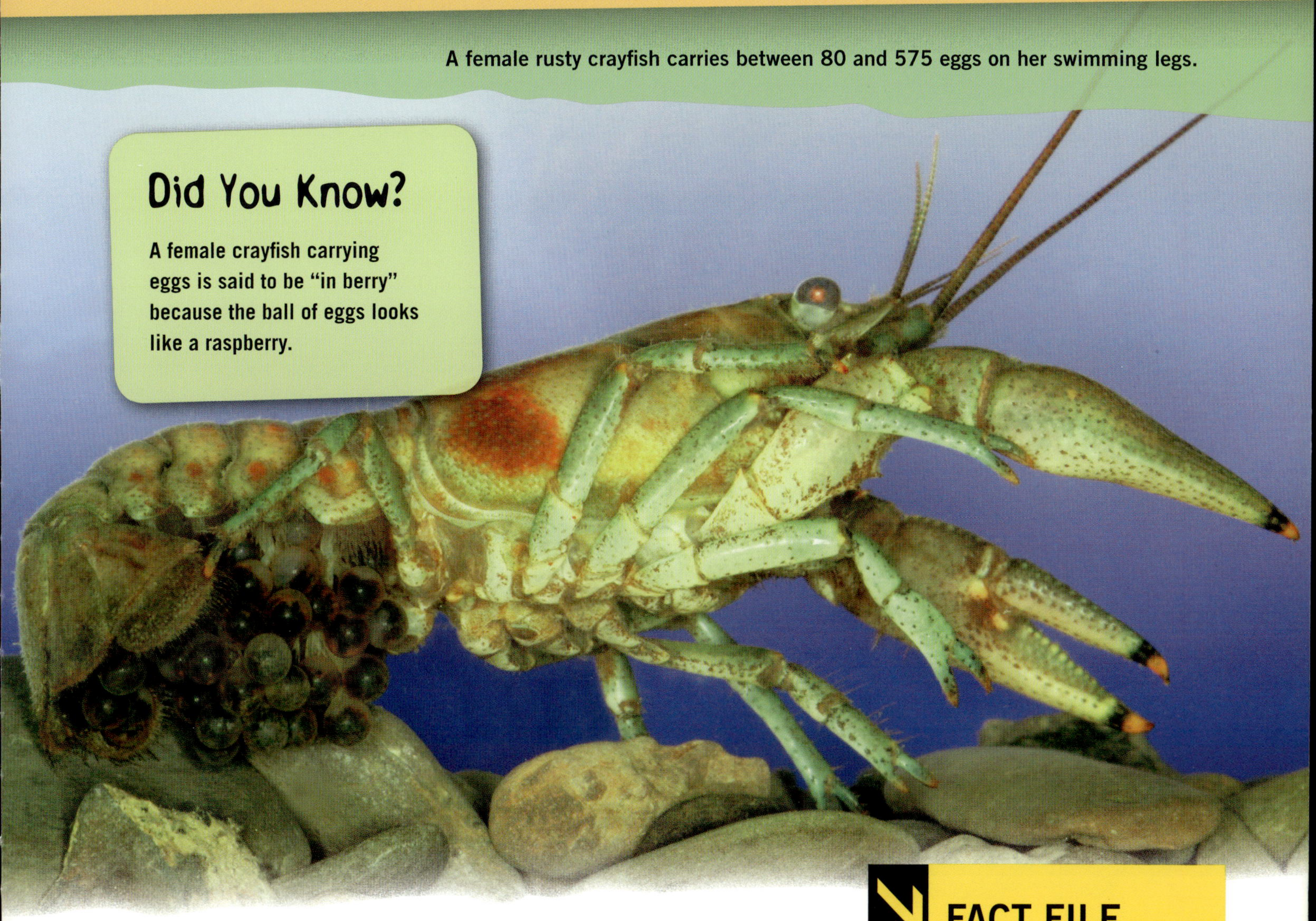

A female rusty crayfish carries between 80 and 575 eggs on her swimming legs.

Did You Know?

A female crayfish carrying eggs is said to be "in berry" because the ball of eggs looks like a raspberry.

FACT FILE

Type of Animal: invertebrate

Length: 1–15.7 inches (2.5–40 cm)

Habitat: streams, ponds, and lakes

Distribution: Europe, Asia, Australia, and North and South America

Number of Eggs: approximately 200

Crayfish

A female crayfish lays eggs. She carries the eggs with her until the young hatch.

A male and a female crayfish mate at breeding time. The female lays eggs several weeks after mating. She attaches the eggs to her swimming legs. After the young hatch from the eggs, they stay with their mother for several weeks.

Keeping Eggs Warm

A female mallard duck sits on her eggs for about four weeks until the ducklings hatch.

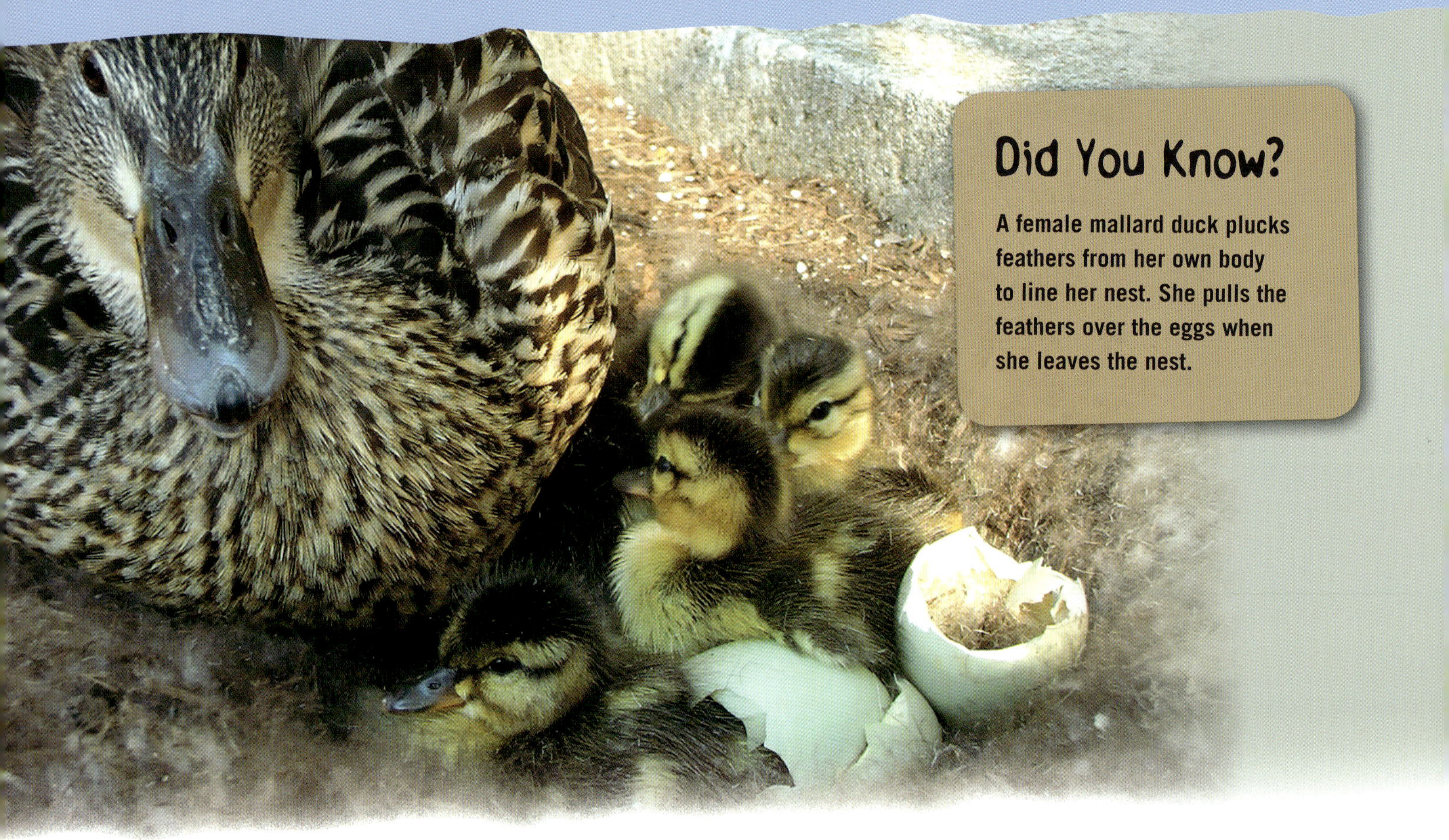

Did You Know?

A female mallard duck plucks feathers from her own body to line her nest. She pulls the feathers over the eggs when she leaves the nest.

FACT FILE

Type of Animal: bird

Length: 1.7–2.2 feet (52–68 cm)

Habitat: rivers, ponds, and lakes

Distribution: Europe, Asia, Australia, and North America

Number of Eggs: 8 to 12

Mallard Duck

A female mallard duck lays oval-shaped, green eggs. She sits on the eggs to keep them warm until the young, called ducklings, hatch.

A male and a female mallard duck mate during the breeding season. The female lays one egg each day in a nest. After she lays the last egg, she sits on all of the eggs, so that all of the ducklings will hatch at about the same time. The ducklings can swim and feed themselves soon after hatching.

Python

A female python lays leathery eggs. She coils around the eggs to keep them warm and to protect them until the young hatch.

A male and a female python mate in the breeding season, and the female lays eggs several weeks later. She basks in the sun or shivers to warm herself, so she can then coil around the eggs and warm them. After hatching, the young pythons care for themselves.

FACT FILE

Type of Animal: reptile

Length: 2–32.8 feet (0.6–10 m)

Habitat: rain forests, forests, woodlands, and deserts

Distribution: Africa, Asia, and Australia

Number of Eggs: 15 to 100

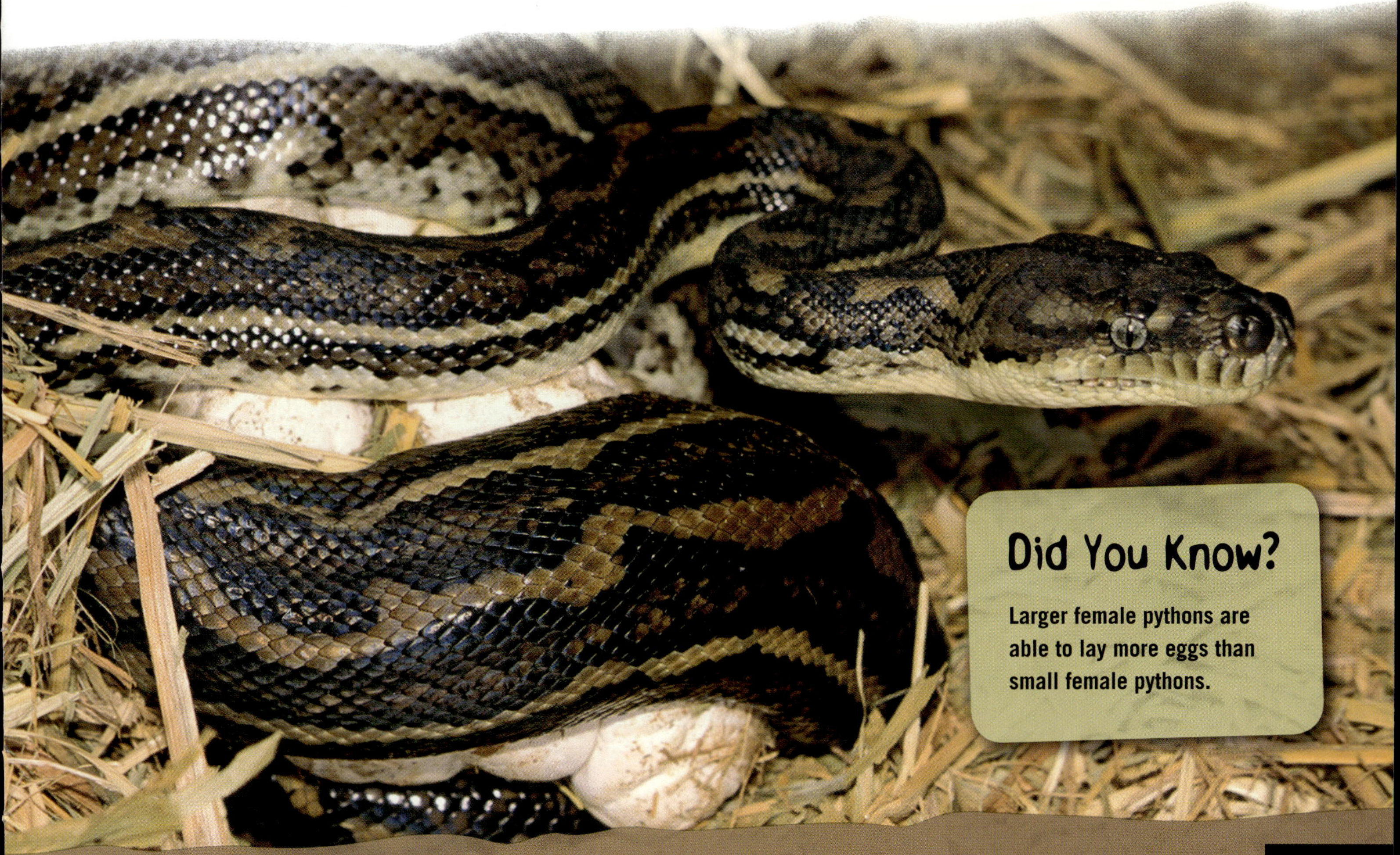

Did You Know?

Larger female pythons are able to lay more eggs than small female pythons.

Female carpet pythons coil around their eggs to keep them warm and guard them from predators.

FACT FILE

Type of Animal: reptile

Length: 5.6–23 feet (1.7–7 m)

Habitat: rivers, lakes, and swamps

Distribution: Africa, Asia, Australia, and North and South America

Number of Eggs: up to 60

Crocodile

A female crocodile lays eggs. She transports the young to water after they hatch from the eggs.

During breeding time, a male and a female crocodile mate. The female lays eggs in a nest about six weeks later. She guards the eggs for approximately 12 weeks, but when she hears the young hatching, she opens up the nest. She carries the young to water in her mouth, and she often guards the young for a few more weeks.

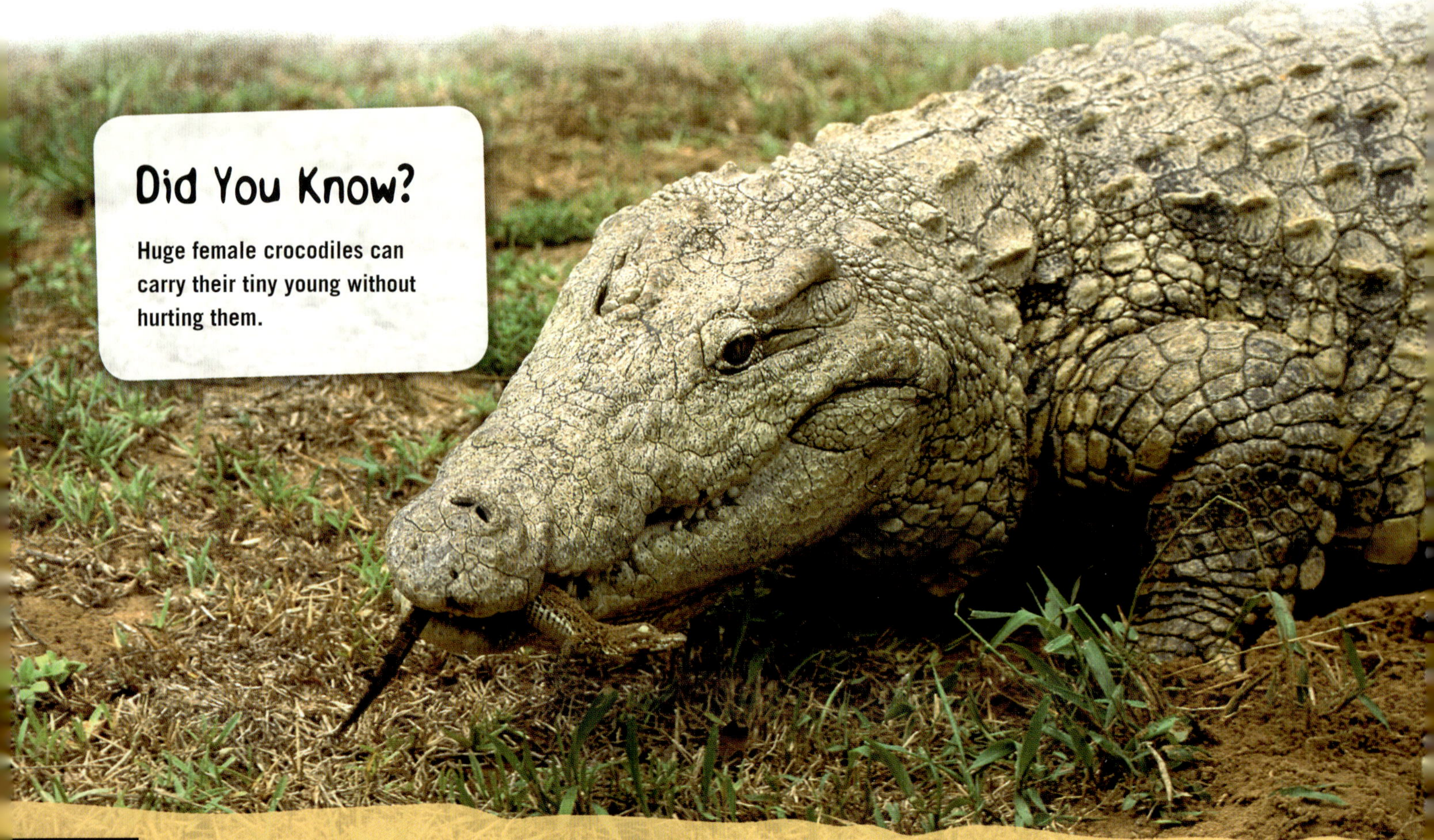

Did You Know?

Huge female crocodiles can carry their tiny young without hurting them.

A newly hatched Nile crocodile is transported to water in its mother's toothy mouth.

Newly hatched animal young are sometimes given a ride to water.

A strawberry poison dart frog transports its young, one tadpole at a time.

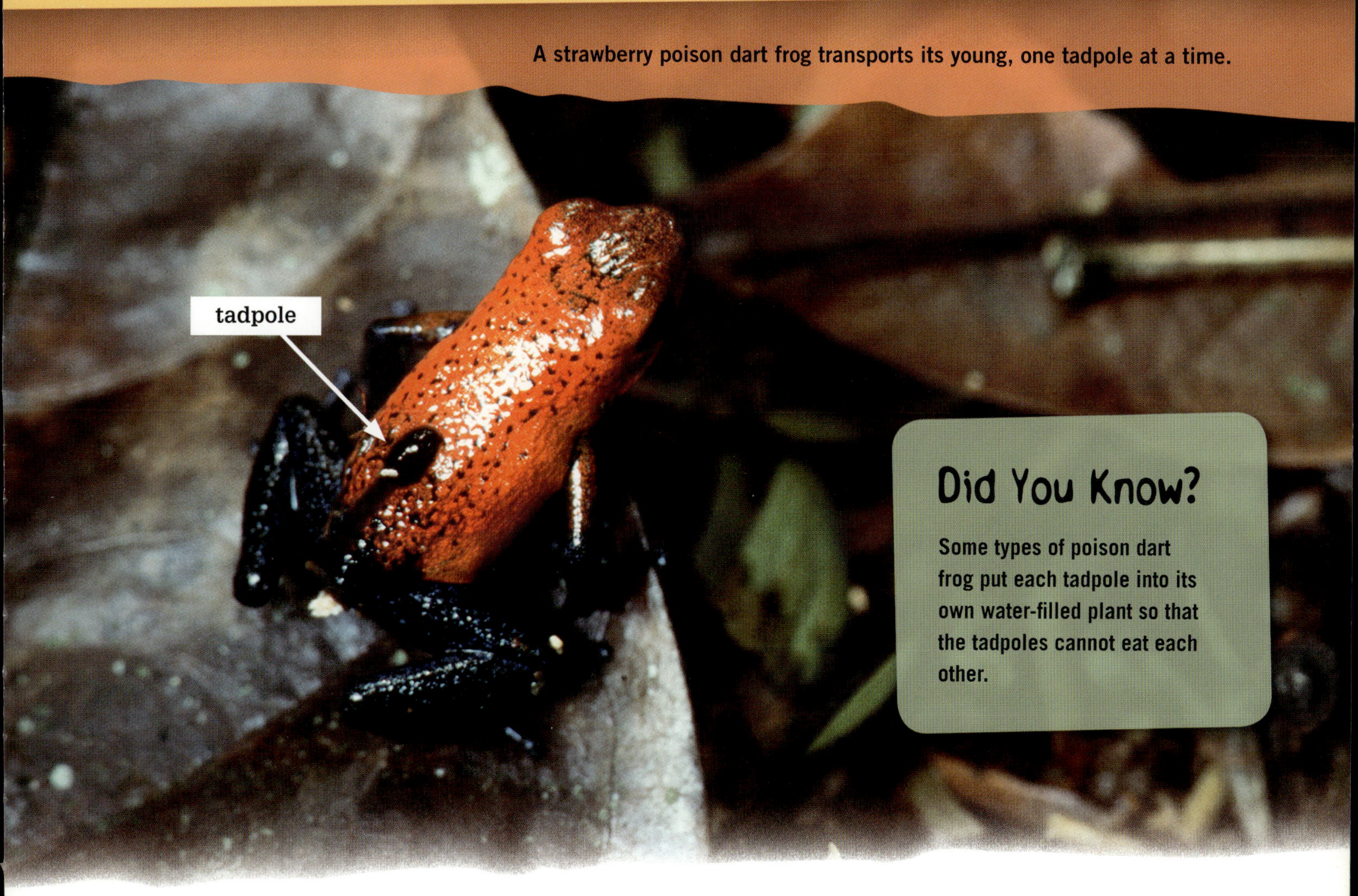

Did You Know?

Some types of poison dart frog put each tadpole into its own water-filled plant so that the tadpoles cannot eat each other.

Poison Dart Frog

A female poison dart frog lays eggs. One parent transports the young, called tadpoles, to water.

The female lays eggs on a plant and the male fertilizes them. One parent guards the eggs until the tadpoles hatch. The tadpoles wriggle onto the parent's back, and the parent carries them to a pond or water-filled plant. Some females lay unfertilized eggs in the water for the tadpoles to eat.

FACT FILE

Type of Animal: amphibian

Length: 0.04–2.4 inches (1–6 cm)

Habitat: rain forests

Distribution: Central and South America

Number of Eggs: 2 to 30

Carrying Young

A female wolf spider sometimes walks around with several layers of spiderlings on her **abdomen**.

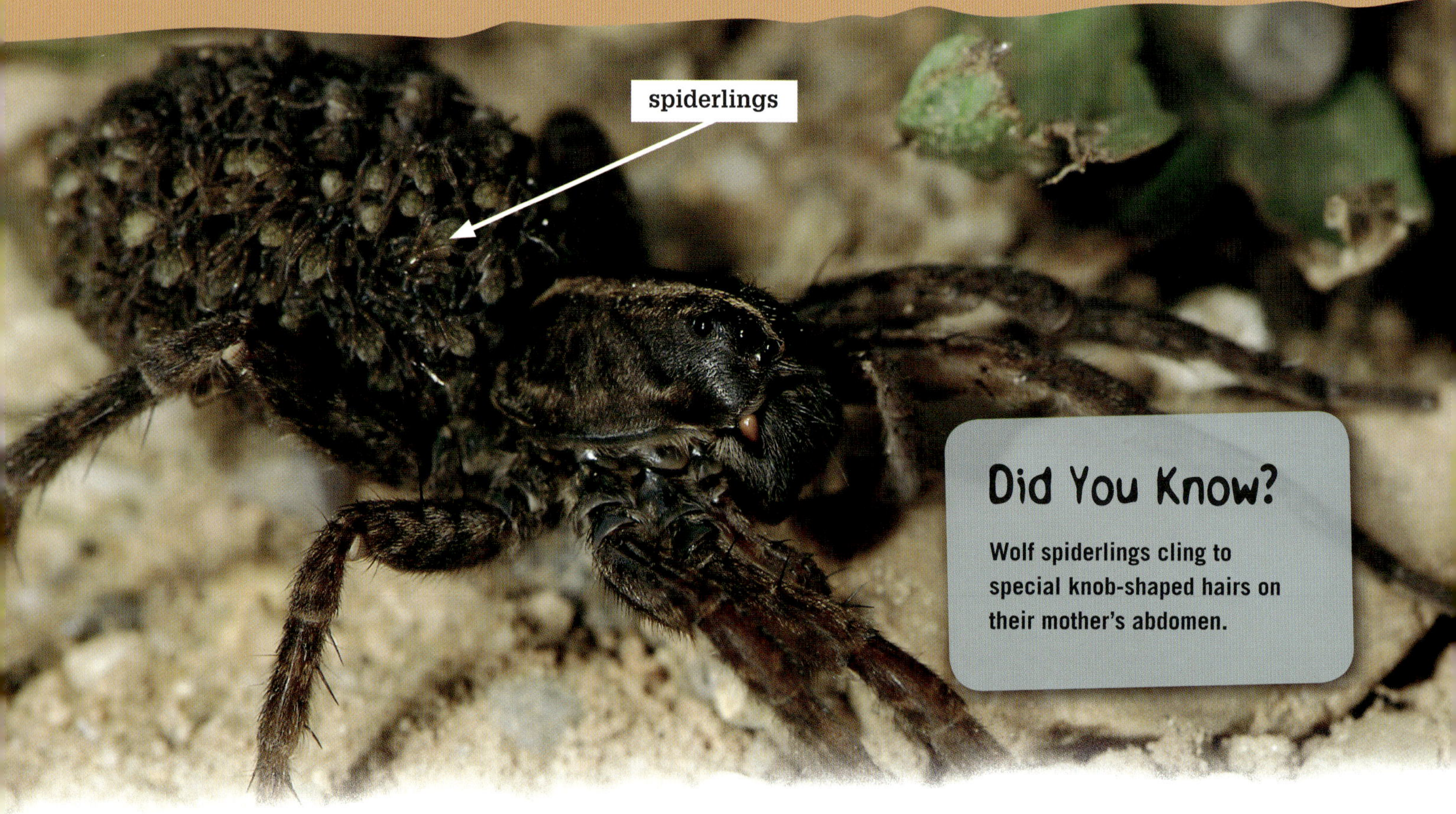

Did You Know?

Wolf spiderlings cling to special knob-shaped hairs on their mother's abdomen.

FACT FILE

Type of Animal: invertebrate

Length: 0.04–1.2 inches (1–30 mm)

Habitat: in grass or under stones, logs, or leaf litter

Distribution: every continent except Antarctica

Number of Eggs: approximately 100

Wolf Spider

A female wolf spider lays eggs and carries them around with her. After they hatch, she carries the young, called spiderlings, on her abdomen for a few days.

A male and a female wolf spider mate, then the female lays eggs. She carries the eggs in a round, silk egg sac attached to her spinnerets. When the spiderlings hatch, they crawl onto their mother's abdomen. They leave their mother when they are able to care for themselves.

Scorpion

A female scorpion gives birth to live young, called scorplings. She carries the scorplings on her back from 1 to 50 days.

A male scorpion grasps a female's **pincers** with his own when he is ready to mate. He releases a packet of sperm and moves the female over it. The female then becomes pregnant. When the scorplings are born, they crawl onto their mother's back. They leave her back after they have shed their outer covering for the first time.

FACT FILE

Type of Animal: invertebrate

Length: approximately 2.4 inches (6 cm)

Habitat: forests, grasslands, and deserts

Distribution: every continent except Antarctica

Number of Young: approximately 25

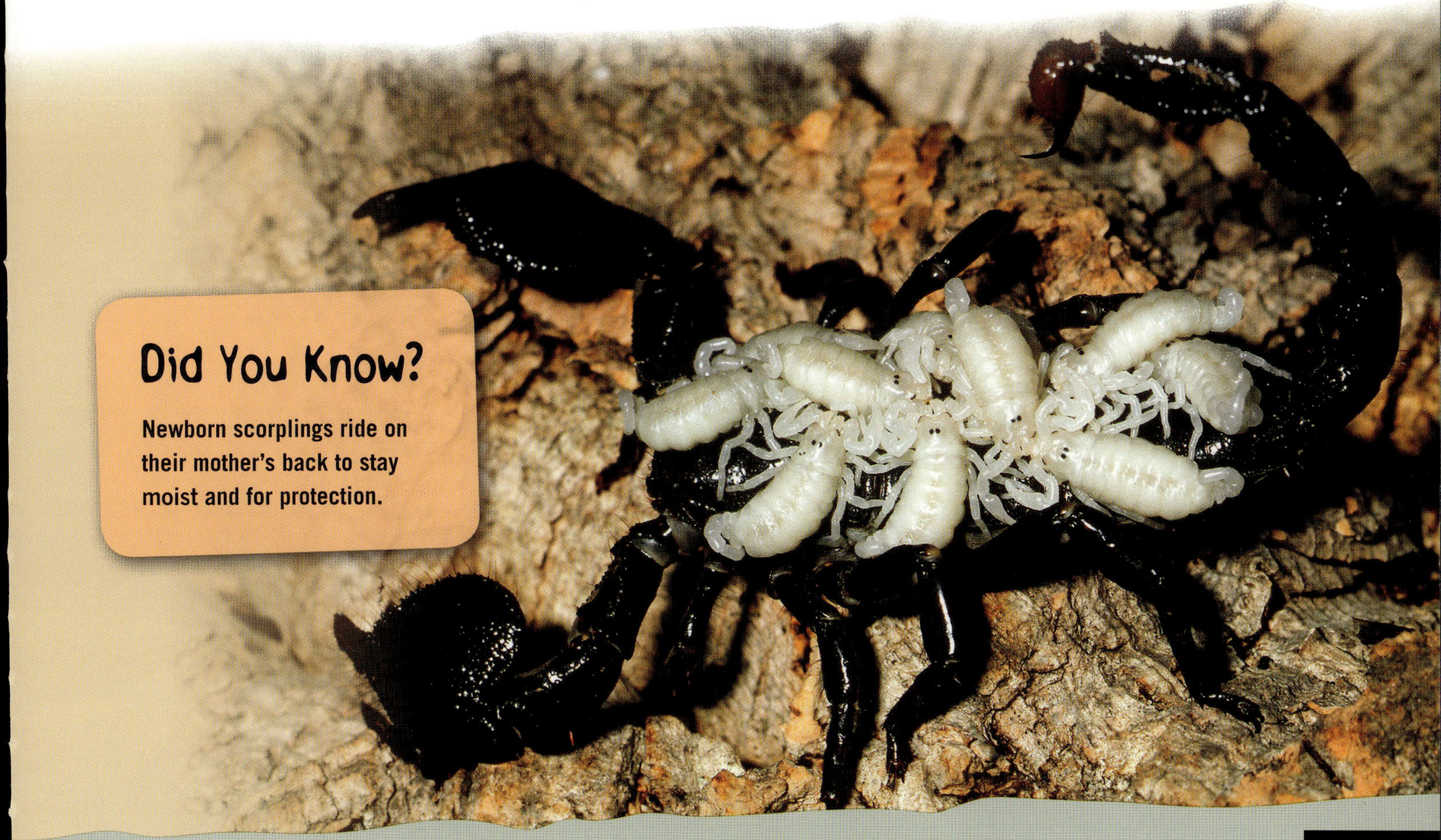

Did You Know?

Newborn scorplings ride on their mother's back to stay moist and for protection.

Newborn emperor scorplings must ride on their mother's back or they will die.

Wallaby

A female wallaby gives birth to one young, called a joey. She carries the joey in a pouch on the front of her body.

A male and a female wallaby mate, and the female becomes pregnant. She gives birth to a joey after 21 to 38 days. The joey crawls into its mother's pouch, attaches itself to a nipple, and drinks milk. It leaves the pouch after three to nine months. It drinks milk for a further one to eight months.

Did You Know?

A female wallaby often cares for one joey in her pouch as well as another, older joey that has left her pouch but still drinks her milk.

FACT FILE

Type of Animal: mammal

Head and Body Length: 1.5–3.4 feet (45–105 cm)

Habitat: rain forests, forests, woodlands, deserts, and rocky hills

Distribution: Australia and New Guinea

Number of Young: 1

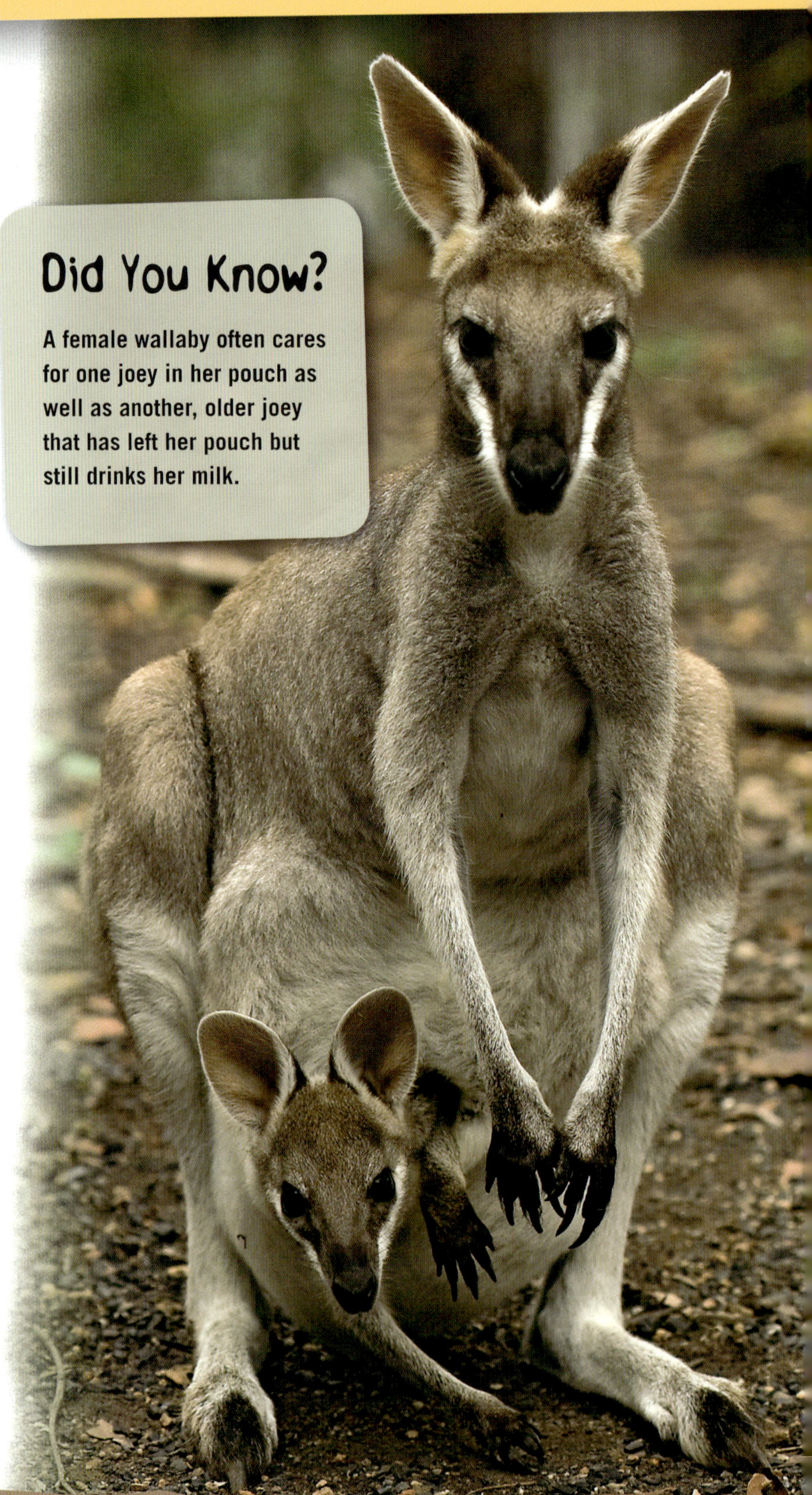

A wallaby joey stays in its mother's pouch for up to ten months.

A pouch protects some young animals as they develop.

The shape of a female marsupial frog's eggs can be seen through the pouch on her back.

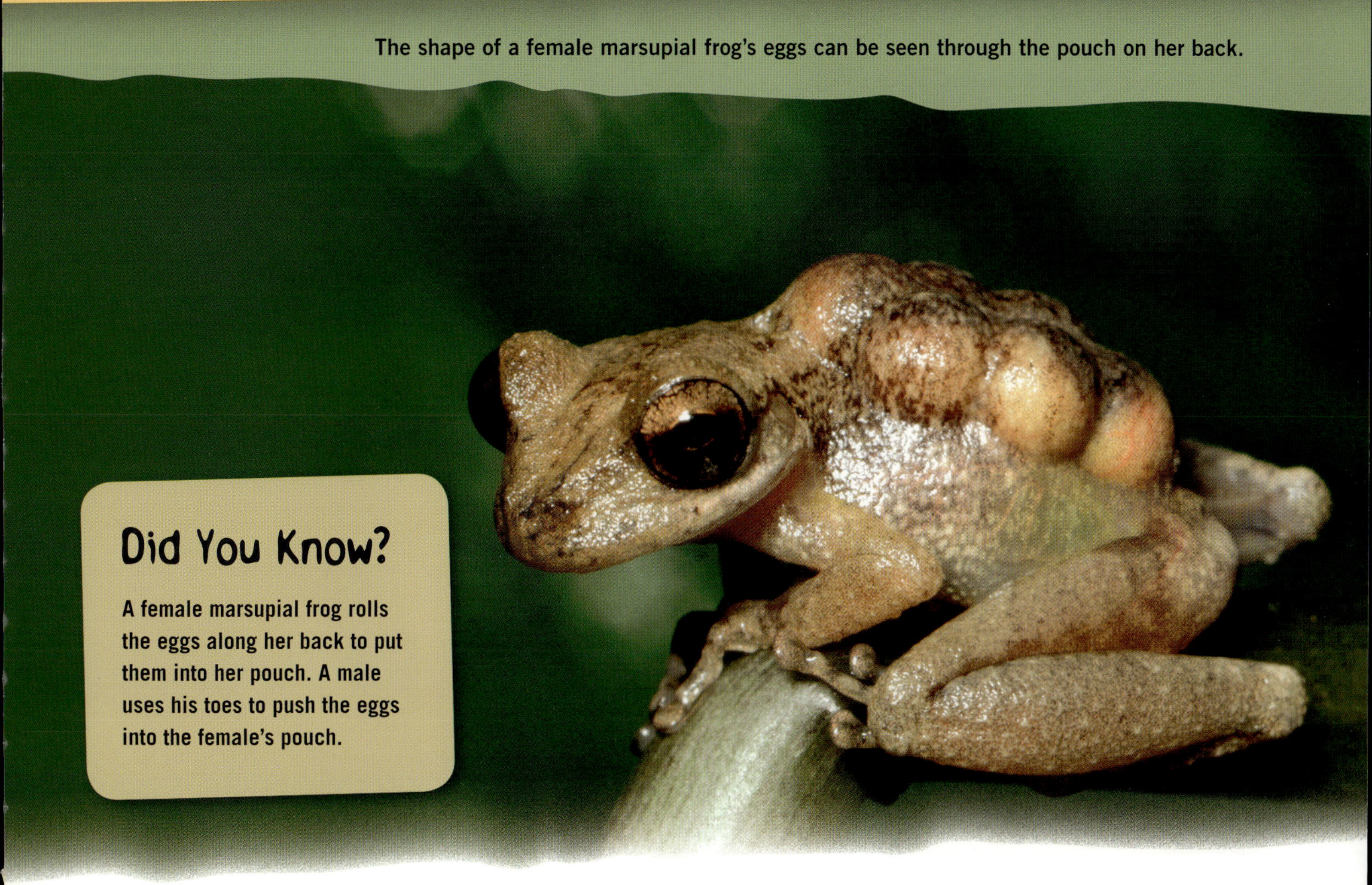

Did You Know?

A female marsupial frog rolls the eggs along her back to put them into her pouch. A male uses his toes to push the eggs into the female's pouch.

Marsupial Frog

A female marsupial frog carries her eggs in a pouch on her back until the tadpoles hatch or the tiny frogs come out.

The female marsupial frog lays eggs, and the male fertilizes them. One parent then puts the eggs into the female's pouch. In some types of marsupial frogs, tadpoles hatch from the eggs, and the female releases them into water. The eggs of other types of marsupial frogs develop into tiny frogs.

FACT FILE

Type of Animal: amphibian

Length: 2–2.8 inches (5–7 cm)

Habitat: rain forests

Distribution: Central and South America

Number of Eggs: approximately 100

Father Care

A male seahorse spends several hours giving birth to his young.

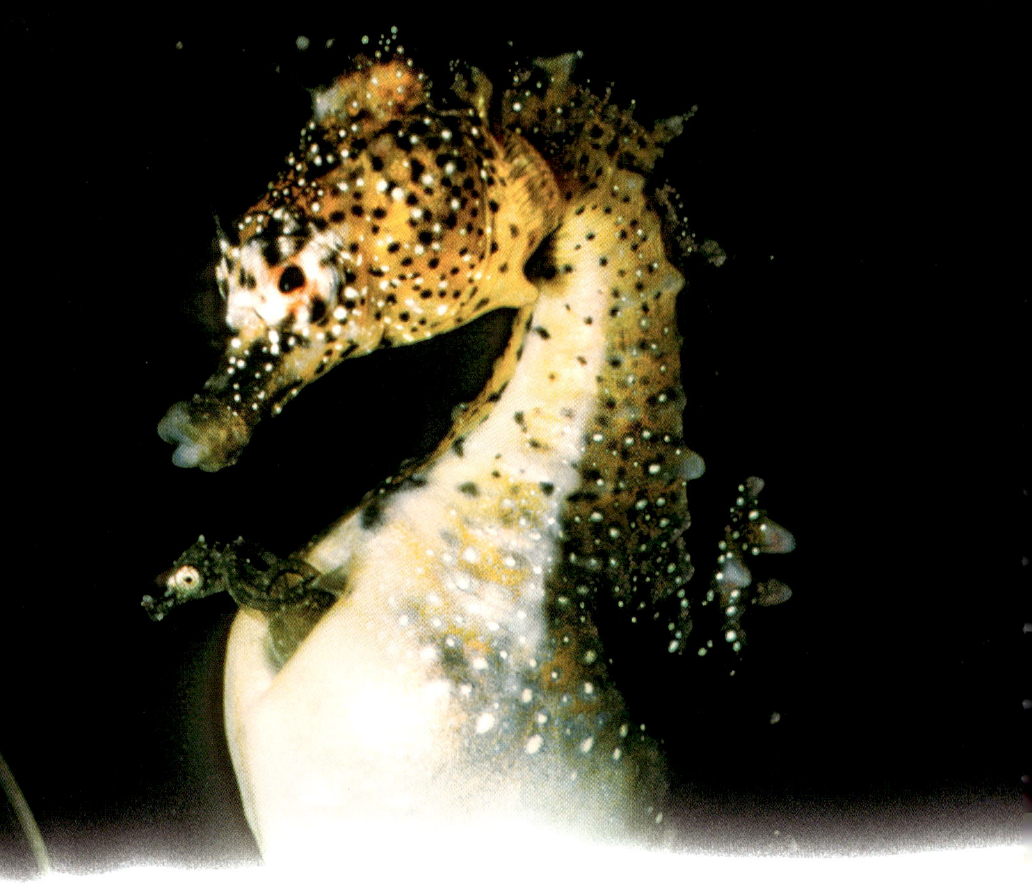

Did You Know?

Seahorses swim together before dawn each day. This helps them be in the best position when the female is ready to lay her eggs.

FACT FILE

Type of Animal: fish

Length: 1.6–11.8 inches (4–30 cm)

Habitat: coral and rocky reefs, sea-grass meadows, and sponge gardens

Distribution: worldwide in warm seas and oceans

Number of Eggs: 100 to 200

Seahorse

A male seahorse gets pregnant! He carries the eggs in a pouch and gives birth to the young.

A female seahorse lays eggs in a male seahorse's pouch. The male then fertilizes the eggs. He protects the eggs until the young hatch, after two to four weeks, then he pushes the young out of his pouch by squeezing his muscles. The young swim away and look after themselves.

Emperor Penguin

A male emperor penguin keeps an egg warm in the bitterly cold Antarctic winter.

A male and a female emperor penguin mate. The female then lays an egg, and the male puts the egg on his feet and covers it with a fold of skin. The female returns to the ocean to eat. The young, called a chick, hatches from the egg after nine weeks. The male gives the chick a little food. When the female returns, the male and female both feed the chick until it can feed itself.

FACT FILE

Type of Animal: bird

Length: 3.3–4.3 feet (100–130 cm)

Habitat: cold oceans and icy land

Distribution: Southern Ocean and Antarctica

Number of Eggs: 1

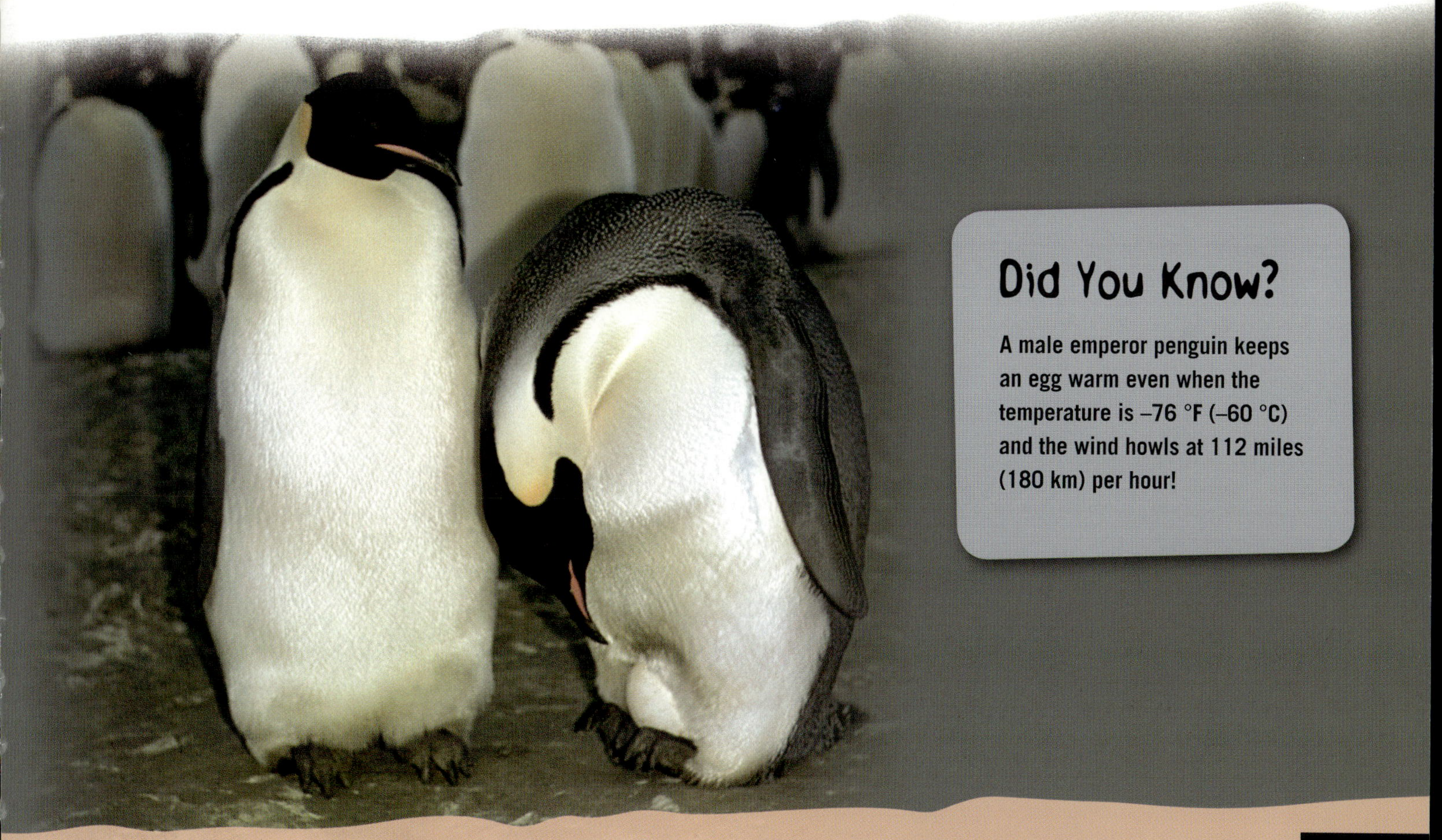

Did You Know?

A male emperor penguin keeps an egg warm even when the temperature is –76 °F (–60 °C) and the wind howls at 112 miles (180 km) per hour!

A male emperor penguin holds an egg on his feet so that it does not freeze on the ice.

FACT FILE

Type of Animal: mammal

Height: 4.5 feet (137 cm)

Habitat: rain forests and forests

Distribution: Borneo and Sumatra

Number of Young: 1

Orangutan

A female orangutan spends most of her adult life caring for her young.

A male and a female orangutan mate, then the male goes away. The female becomes pregnant and gives birth to one young after eight to nine months. The young clings to its mother's chest or back and drinks her milk. It stays with its mother for at least six years.

Did You Know?

A female orangutan teaches her young to find food, swing through the trees, and make a nest in which to sleep.

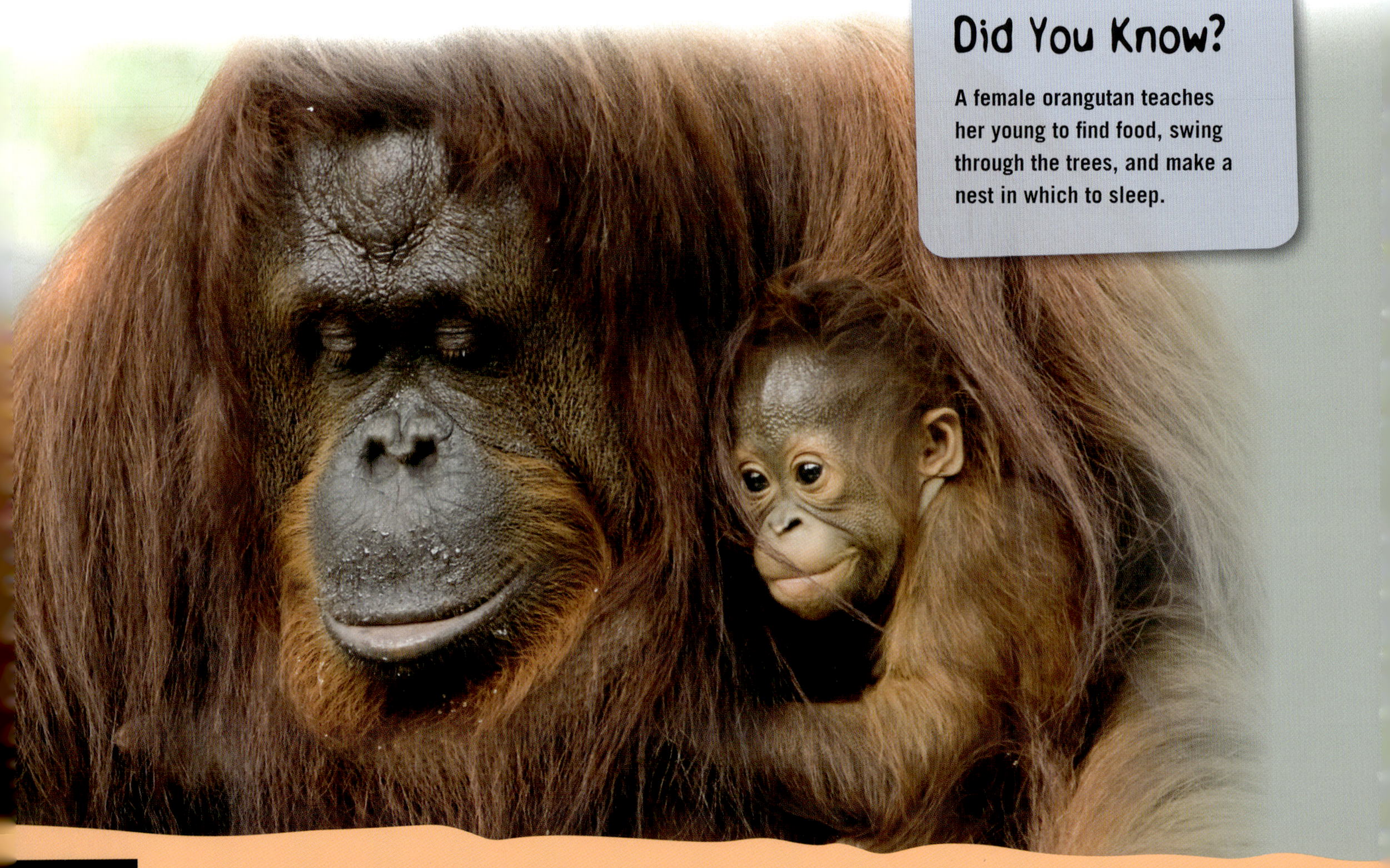

A female orangutan feeds, protects, and transports her young.

Some mothers look after their young without any help from the fathers.

A tigress raises her cubs alone.

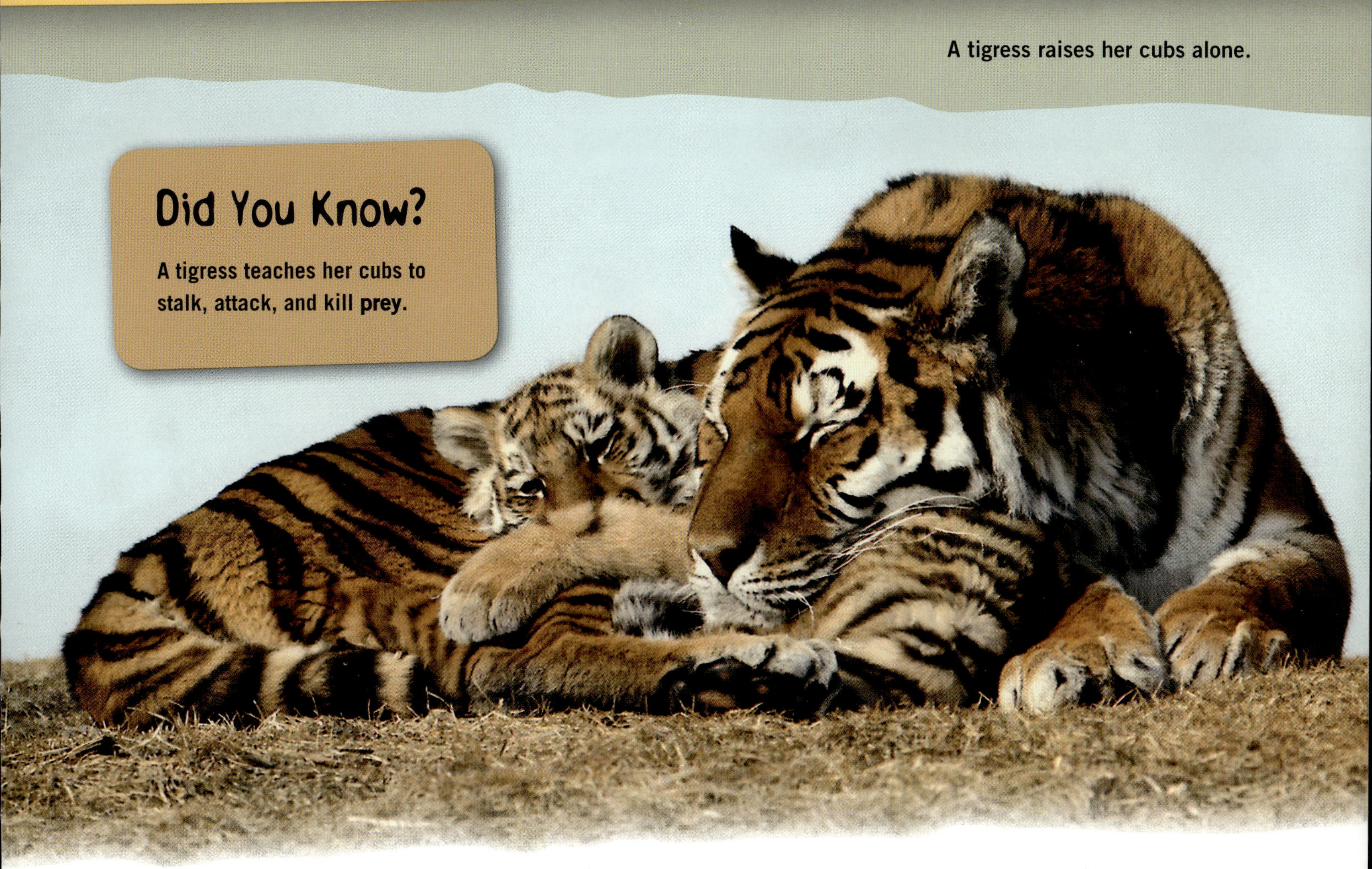

Did You Know?

A tigress teaches her cubs to stalk, attack, and kill **prey**.

Tiger

A female tiger, called a tigress, feeds, cares for, and protects her young, called cubs.

A tiger and a tigress mate at any time of the year. The tiger leaves after mating, and the tigress becomes pregnant. After about four months, she gives birth to the cubs. The cubs drink their mother's milk. They stay with their mother until they are between 18 months and 3 years old, and can hunt on their own.

FACT FILE

Type of Animal: mammal

Head and Body Length: 7.2 feet (2.2 m)

Habitat: forests, grasslands, and mangrove swamps

Distribution: Asia

Number of Young: usually 2 or 3

Two-parent Care

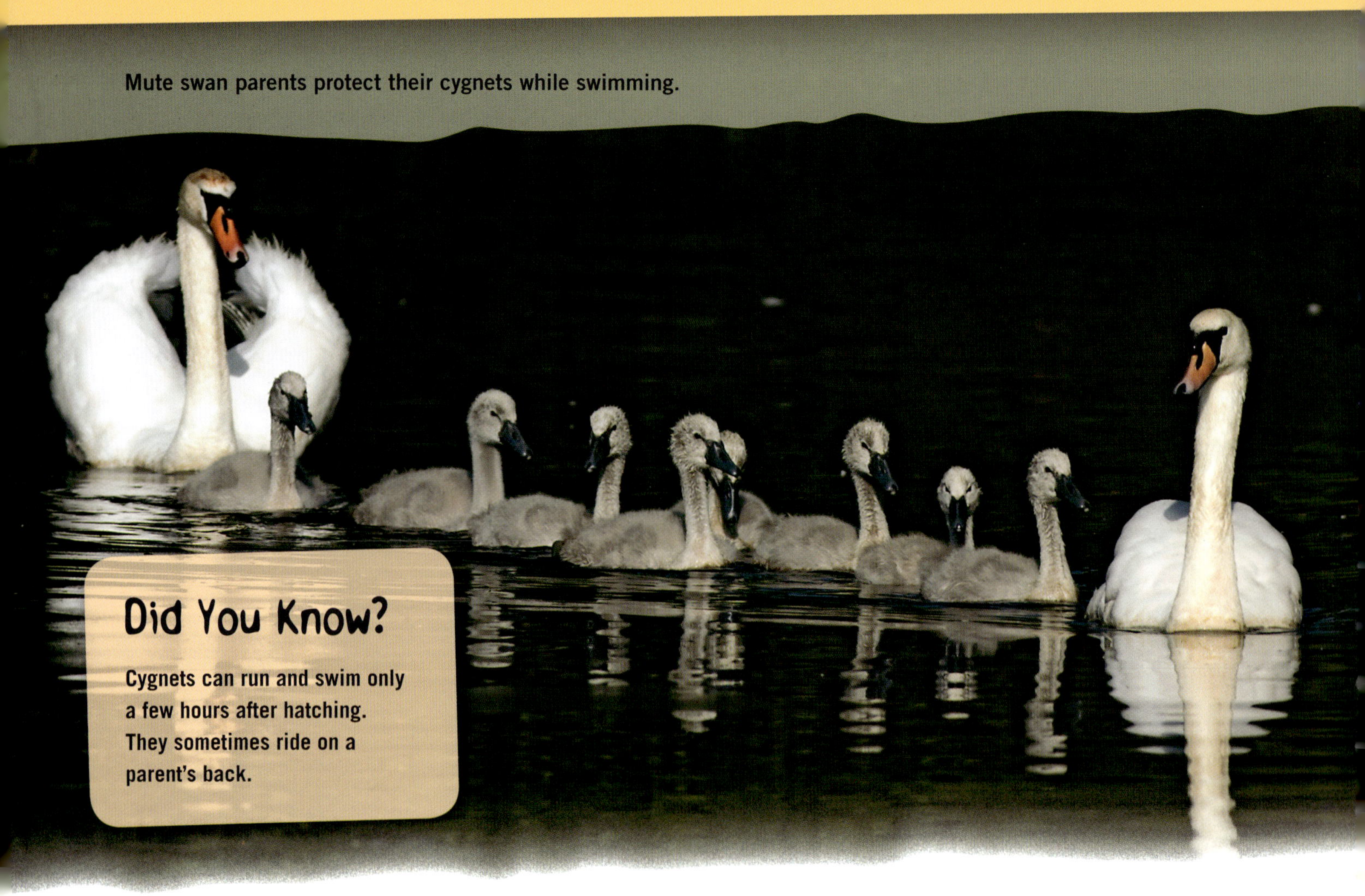

Mute swan parents protect their cygnets while swimming.

Did You Know?

Cygnets can run and swim only a few hours after hatching. They sometimes ride on a parent's back.

FACT FILE

Type of Animal: bird

Length: 4.3–5.2 feet (1.3–1.6 m)

Habitat: ponds, lakes, and rivers

Distribution: Europe and Asia

Number of Eggs: 3 to 11

Mute Swan

Mute swans form pairs for life. Both parents keep the eggs warm and protect the young, called cygnets.

A male and a female mute swan mate during the breeding season. The female lays eggs in a nest of plants on the ground. The cygnets hatch after 35 days. They leave the nest after one or two days but stay with their parents for several months.

In some family groups, parents stay together to warm their eggs and raise their young.

Flamingo

Both flamingo parents keep their egg warm and feed the young, called a chick.

A male and a female flamingo mate after good rainfalls. The female lays an egg in a cone-shaped nest made of mud, and the chick hatches after about one month. Both parents feed the chick a milky substance they make in their bodies. The chick leaves the nest after about five days, but the parents feed and protect it for about three months.

FACT FILE

Type of Animal: bird

Height: 3–4.9 feet (90–150 cm)

Habitat: lakes, lagoons, and coasts

Distribution: Africa, Europe, Asia, and South America

Number of Eggs: 1

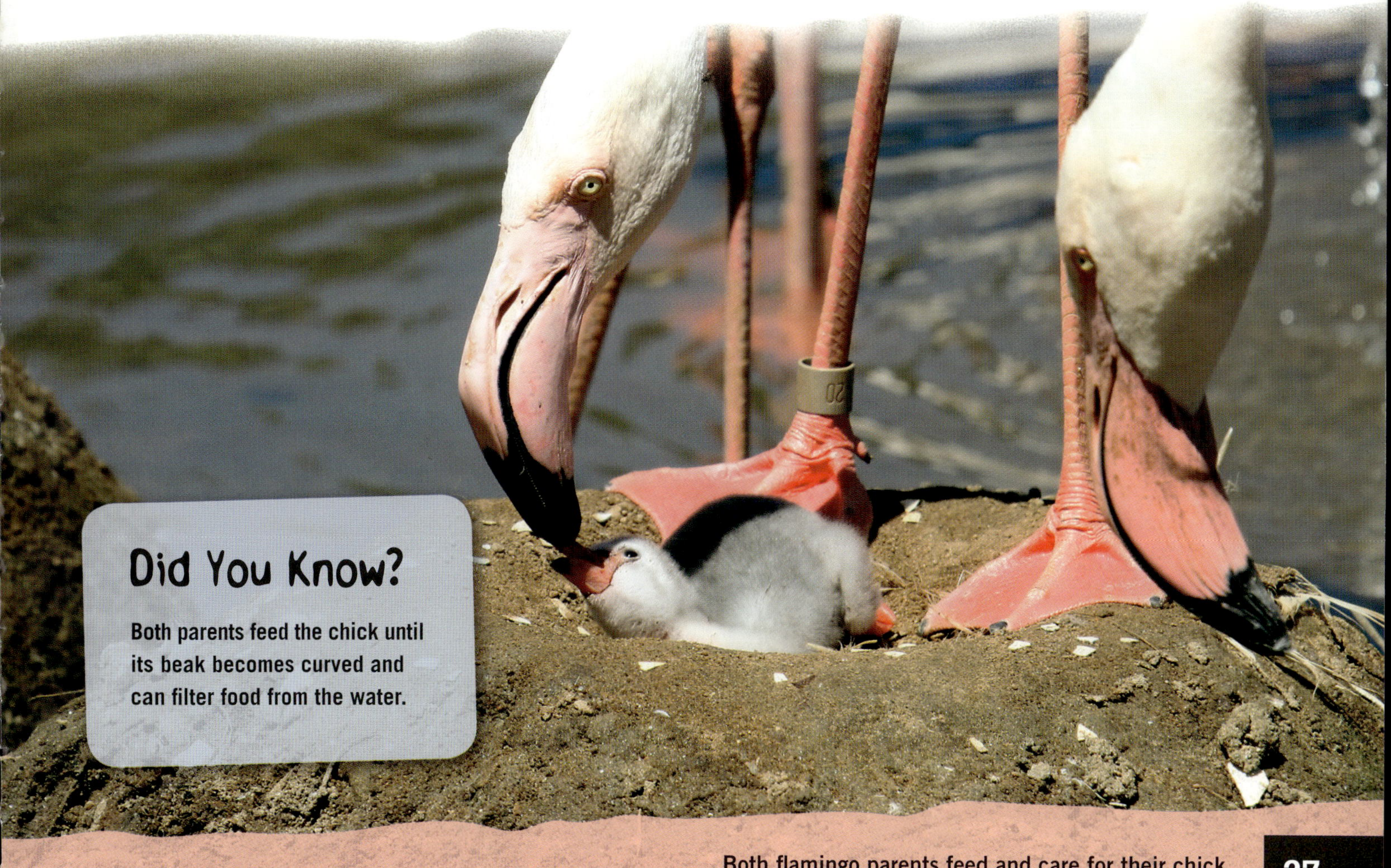

Did You Know?

Both parents feed the chick until its beak becomes curved and can filter food from the water.

Both flamingo parents feed and care for their chick.

FACT FILE

Type of Animal: mammal

Head and Body Length: 4.9–6.9 feet (1.5–2.1 m)

Habitat: woodlands and grasslands

Distribution: Africa and Asia

Number of Young: usually 2 to 4

Lion

All lions in a pride breed at the same time. The female lions, called lionesses, help each other raise the young, called cubs.

A lion and a lioness mate, and the lioness becomes pregnant. About four months later, she gives birth to the cubs in a den. She feeds the cubs milk. She takes the cubs to join the pride when they are about six weeks old. If she goes away hunting, one of the other lionesses will feed her cubs milk.

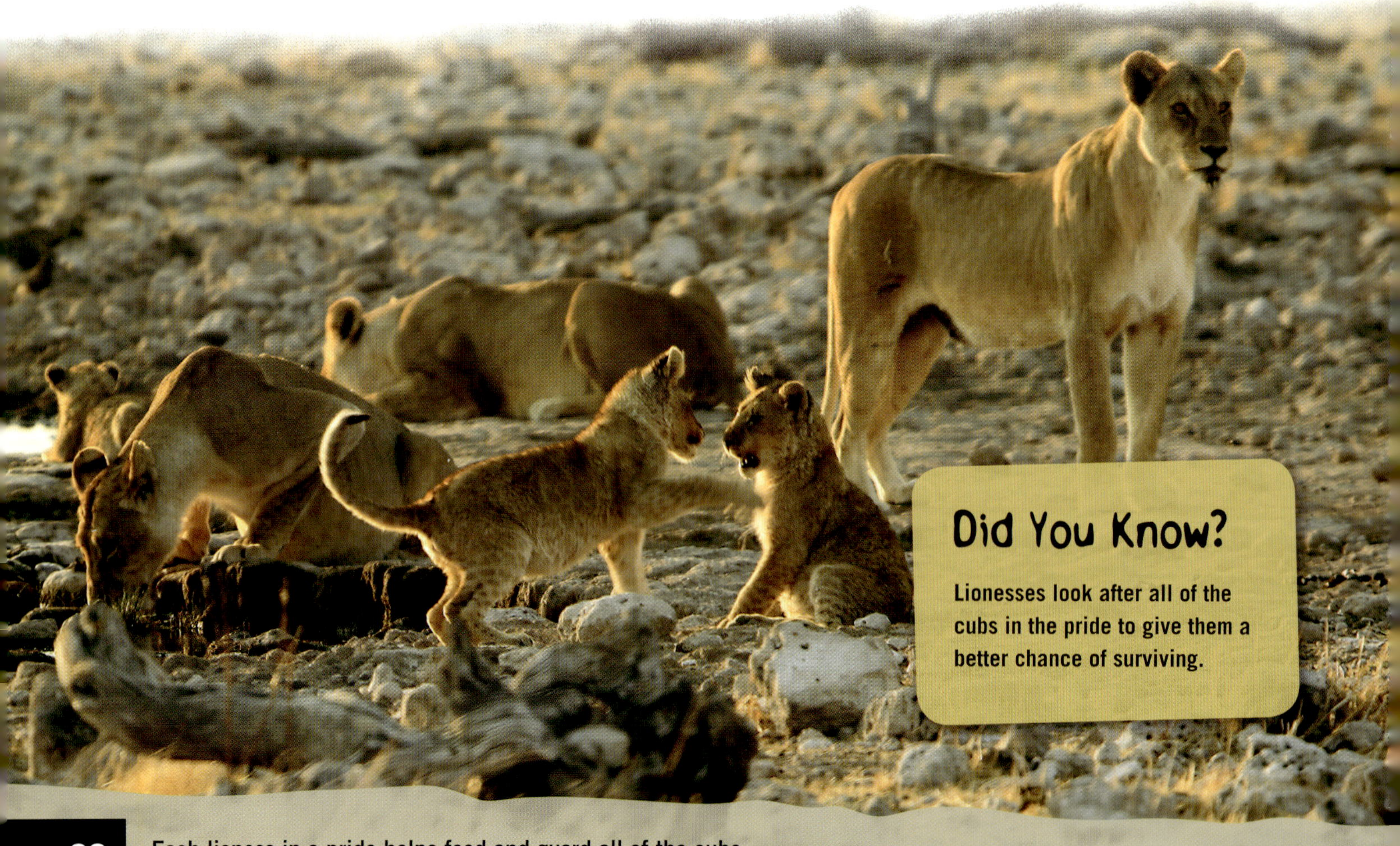

Did You Know?

Lionesses look after all of the cubs in the pride to give them a better chance of surviving.

Each lioness in a pride helps feed and guard all of the cubs.

All of the elephants in a family group help keep the calves safe while drinking.

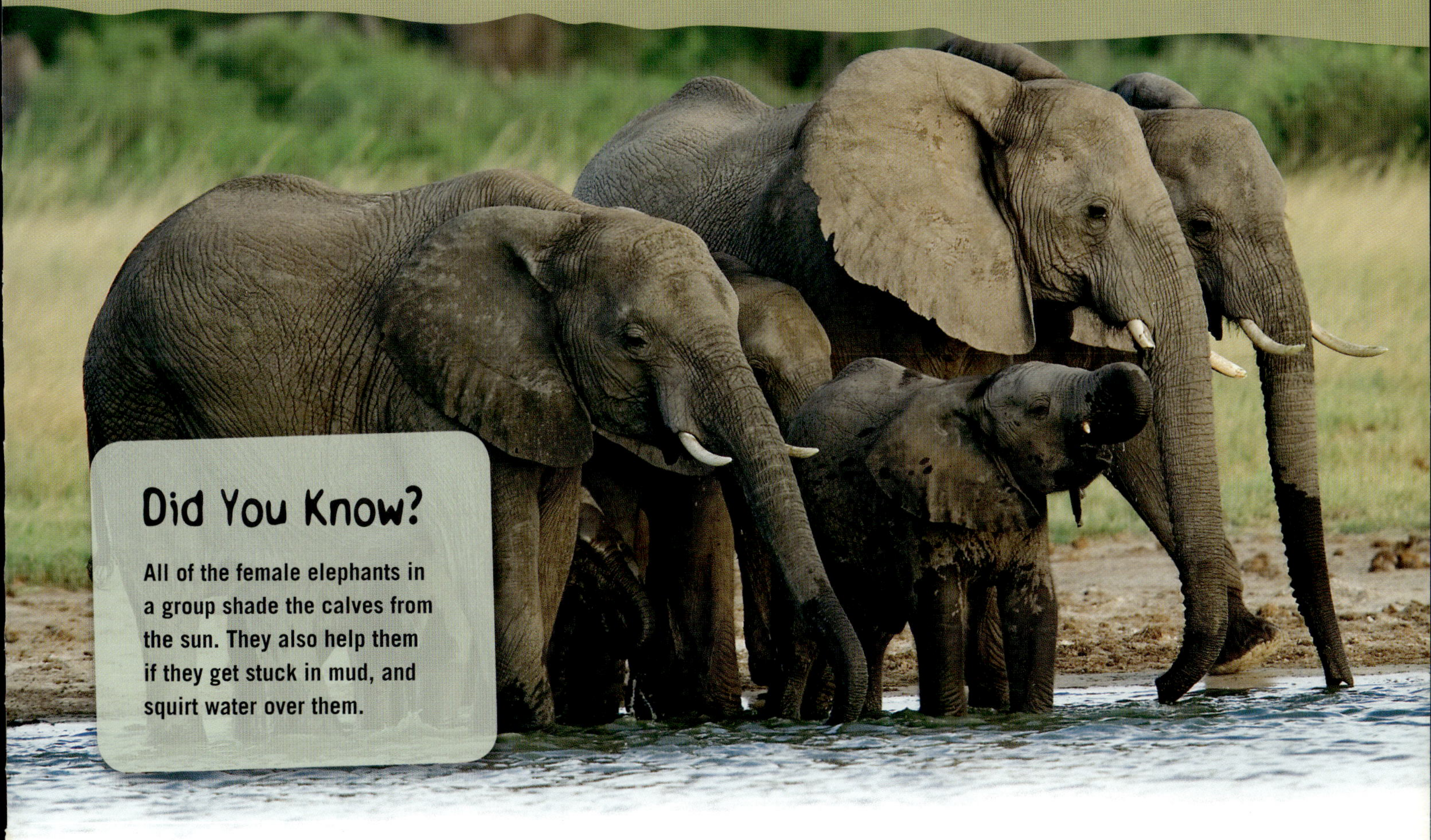

Did You Know?

All of the female elephants in a group shade the calves from the sun. They also help them if they get stuck in mud, and squirt water over them.

Elephant

Female elephants live in family groups. They all help raise and protect the young, called calves.

A male and a female elephant mate, and the female becomes pregnant. A calf is born 22 months later. When it is born, all of the elephants in the group gather around the calf and touch it with their trunks. The calf drinks its mother's milk for two to three years. It receives help and protection from all of the other elephants.

FACT FILE

Type of Animal: mammal

Height at Shoulder: 9.8–13.1 feet (3–4 m)

Habitat: rain forests, forests, woodlands, and grasslands

Distribution: Africa and Asia

Number of Young: 1

Believe It or Not:

Foster Parents

A cuckoo baby is much larger than its **foster parent**—and very hungry!

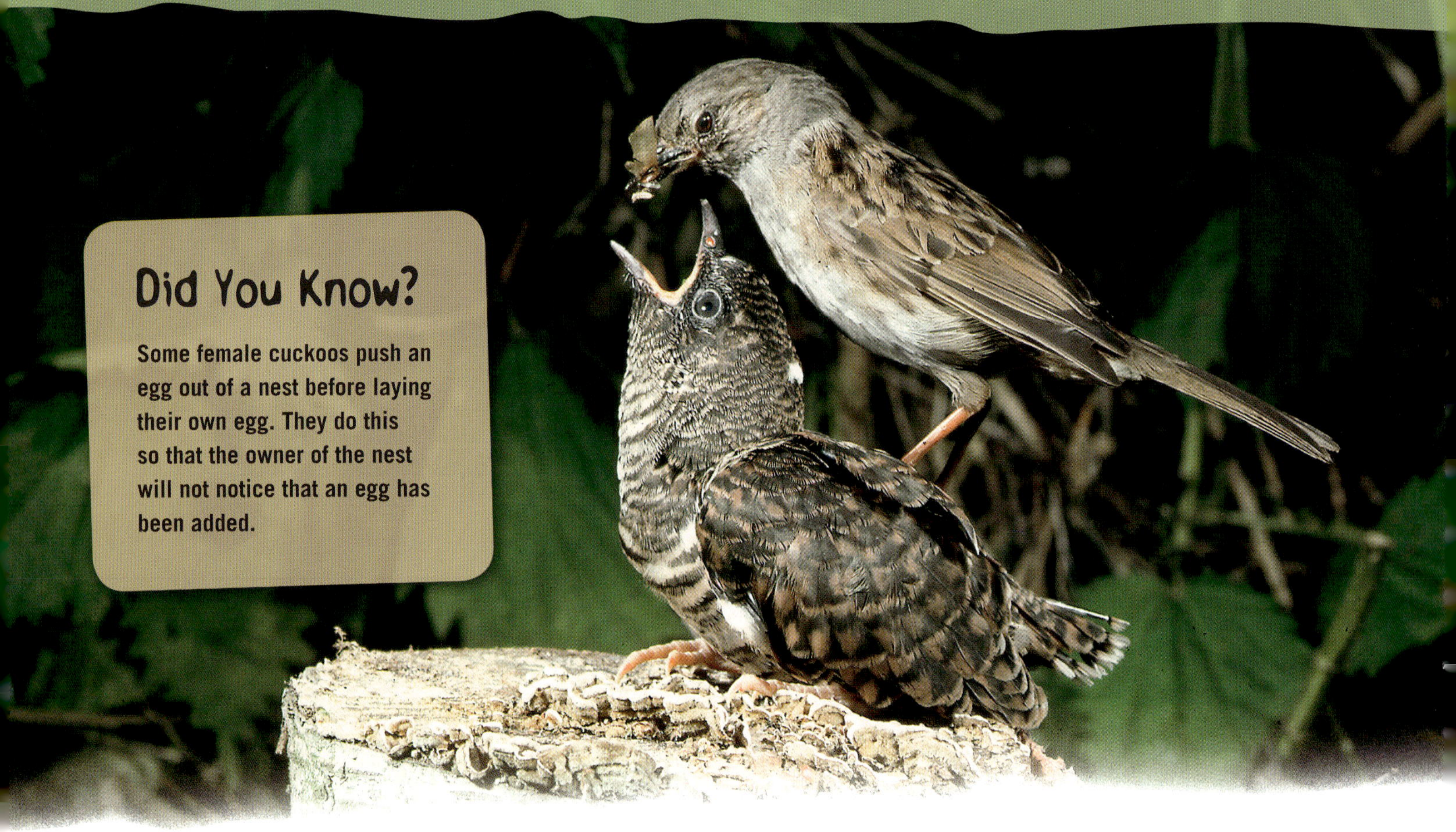

Did You Know?

Some female cuckoos push an egg out of a nest before laying their own egg. They do this so that the owner of the nest will not notice that an egg has been added.

FACT FILE

Type of Animal: bird

Length: 6.3–35.4 inches (16–90 cm)

Habitat: rain forests, forests, and woodlands

Distribution: every continent except Antarctica

Number of Eggs: 1 per nest

Cuckoo

Many types of cuckoos lay eggs in the nests of other birds. They let the other birds, the foster parents, keep their eggs warm and raise their young.

A male and a female cuckoo mate in the breeding season. The female then lays an egg in the nest of a different type of bird. The cuckoo's egg looks like the other bird's eggs. When the young cuckoo hatches from the egg, it pushes the foster parent's eggs and young out of the nest so it can eat all of the food.

Glossary

abdomen the back part of an insect's or spider's body

amphibian an animal that spends the first part of its life living in water and the second part of its life living on land

breeding having young

currents the steady flow of water in a certain direction

fertilize to make an egg able to develop into a new individual

foster parent a parent who cares for young that do not belong to them

invertebrate an animal without a backbone

litters groups of young animals born at the same time

mammal an animal that feeds its young with its own milk

marsupial an animal that keeps its young in a pouch

moisture dampness

oxygen a gas that is part of the air we breathe

pincers small claws

predators animals that hunt and kill other animals for food

prey animals that are hunted and caught for food by other animals

pride a group of lions

reptile a creeping or crawling animal that is covered with scales

sperm a male cell that can join with a female cell, called an ovum, to develop into a new individual

spinnerets organs in a spider's body that make silk

unfertilized cannot produce young animals

Index